RETRAINING
the BRAIN

RETRAINING the BRAIN

Applied Neuroscience in Exposure Therapy for PTSD

Sheila A. M. Rauch and Carmen P. McLean

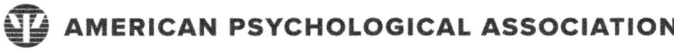 AMERICAN PSYCHOLOGICAL ASSOCIATION

Published by
American Psychological Association
750 First Street, NE
Washington, DC 20002
https://www.apa.org

Order Department
https://www.apa.org/pubs/books
order@apa.org

In the U.K., Europe, Africa, and the Middle East, copies may be ordered from Eurospan
https://www.eurospanbookstore.com/apa
info@eurospangroup.com

Typeset in Charter and Interstate by TIPS Technical Publishing, Inc., Carrboro, NC
Printer: Sheridan Books, Chelsea, MI
Cover Designer: Nicci Falcone, Potomac, MD

Library of Congress Cataloging-in-Publication Data
Names: Rauch, Sheila A. M., author. | McLean, Carmen P., author.
Title: Retraining the brain : applied neuroscience in exposure therapy for PTSD / by Sheila
    A.M. Rauch and Carmen P. McLean.
Description: Washington, DC : American Psychological Association, [2021] | Includes biblio-
    graphical references and index.
Identifiers: LCCN 2020048746 (print) | LCCN 2020048747 (ebook) | ISBN 9781433834042
    (paperback) | ISBN 9781433837081 (ebook)
Subjects: LCSH: Post-traumatic stress disorder—Treatment. | Cognitive therapy. |
    Neurosciences.
Classification: LCC RC552.P67 R384 2021 (print) | LCC RC552.P67 (ebook) | DDC
    616.85/21—dc23
LC record available at https://lccn.loc.gov/2020048746
LC ebook record available at https://lccn.loc.gov/2020048747

https://doi.org/10.1037/0000242-000

Printed in the United States of America

10 9 8 7 6 5 4 3 2 1

To all the people with PTSD whom I have known and worked with over my life, your strength, struggle, survival, and willingness to talk with me about the darkest times in your lives form the foundation of this book. To my family, your support is my fuel.

—SHEILA A. M. RAUCH

Thank you to my many brilliant colleagues for inspiring me with your curiosity, determination, and passion. Thank you to my family for helping me keep everything in perspective. Most of all, thank you to those who sought help for PTSD, whose questions and experiences shaped my understanding of how people recover. To those who participate in research, your selfless contribution to science improves our ability to help others overcome PTSD.

—CARMEN P. McLEAN

Contents

Preface

Posttraumatic stress disorder (PTSD) is a debilitating disorder linked with significant mental and physical health comorbidities and impairments in work, social, and family functioning. Fortunately, the past 20 years has seen exponential growth in research focused on PTSD development and treatment and important advances in our understanding of the psychological and neurological processes involved. Notably, most PTSD research to date remains solidly anchored in either neurobiology or psychological methods, with very few studies examining both simultaneously. For our field to take the next leaps in understanding, researchers and clinicians informed by research must learn to integrate research across neurobiology and psychology. *Retraining the Brain: Applied Neuroscience in Exposure Therapy for PTSD* aims to facilitate this integration by providing a primer for mental health clinicians who treat PTSD to connect the constructs involved in effective PTSD treatment with relevant neuroscience research developments. Although several effective treatment options are well established for PTSD, including both medications and trauma-focused psychotherapies, this book focuses on prolonged exposure (PE) therapy for PTSD (Foa et al., 2019). We have chosen to focus on PE because it has been extensively researched in treatment studies as well as mechanistic trials. As a first-line PTSD treatment, PE has also been widely disseminated within the United States and internationally, including use in Japan, China, Israel, across Europe, and in many other countries (Foa, Gillihan, et al., 2013). While some of the findings discussed may be relevant to multiple psychotherapies or medications, space limitations will not allow us to touch on all the possible connections relevant to all possible PTSD treatments.

Part I begins with a review of PE and relevant theory and research to ensure common understanding. In Part II, readers are presented with a neuroscience primer. This section includes terms and processes from neuroscience that may be new to many readers. These chapters, along with the glossary, can be used as a reference for readers as they move through the book. Part III then applies neuroscience constructs and research to the implementation of each primary PE component. Finally, Part IV looks to promising strategies for PE augmentation and developing models of care for people suffering from PTSD with an eye toward improving therapy access, effectiveness/efficacy, efficiency, and engagement.

Of importance, the intersecting impacts of race, gender, and socioeconomic status on the development of PTSD and response to treatment are gaining critical research momentum and may help us to understand some of the heterogeneity we currently see in PTSD. McClendon et al. (2020) provided three key conclusions in their review of the impact of race on PTSD treatment: (a) more rigorous study of the influence of race on outcomes is needed; (b) the majority of the available research supports efficacy across racial or ethnic groups, though differences in magnitude of response to PTSD treatment are also apparent; and (c) treatment initiation and retention may be lower in Black/African American and Hispanic/Latinx groups. The individualized PE protocol makes it amenable for culturally competent clinicians to use in diverse populations, and further examination of outcomes is warranted (Benuto et al., 2020). Although a comprehensive review of this research is beyond the scope of the current book, we emphasize relevant findings when available. In addition, we highlight the use of PE across cultures.

The intention of *Retraining the Brain* is not to make readers neuroscience experts but to build their neuroscience muscles so that they can use the fruits of neuroscience to continuously improve their practice in the treatment of PTSD. While our primary audience is PTSD treatment providers, we also expect that neuroscience researchers may find this book a useful resource to help them understand the psychological theories and processes involved in effective exposure treatment for PTSD. Through this book, we provide a shared understanding that can support discussion between neuroscience and psychological researchers and clinicians and advance new research that takes advantage of the advances in both fields. We hope that this book spurs thought on ways to move research forward and improve clinical care and training of researchers and providers.

PART I THEORY AND OVERVIEW OF PROLONGED EXPOSURE

1 THEORY AND PROLONGED EXPOSURE

Ivan Pavlov's (1849–1936) foundational work on *classical conditioning* demonstrated how a neutral stimulus could come to evoke a response after being paired with a stimulus that naturally evokes a response. Other researchers expanded on this work and established principles such as stimulus generalization, extinction, and spontaneous recovery that have important implications for understanding posttraumatic stress disorder (PTSD).

EARLY LEARNING THEORIES

A basic assumption of the Pavlovian model is that *associative learning* underlies both the development and treatment of excessive fear. In the application of this model to PTSD, the traumatic event is considered an unconditioned stimulus, which has become associated with a variety of nonthreatening conditioned stimuli (e.g., smells, sights, sounds, people). When an association between neutral stimuli and the traumatic event is formed in memory, later exposure to the neutral stimuli activates the representation of the trauma, triggering a fear response, including reexperiencing symptoms, physiological reactivity, and avoidance behavior.

https://doi.org/10.1037/0000242-001
Retraining the Brain: Applied Neuroscience in Exposure Therapy for PTSD,
by S. A. M. Rauch and C. P. McLean

In addition to classical conditioning, B. F. Skinner (1904–1990) is credited with developing the theory of *operant conditioning*, which asserts that behaviors increase or decrease in frequency based on the consequences of the behavior. His work also identified schedules of reinforcement and the processes of shaping, stimulus discrimination, and extinction. Operant conditioning is highly relevant to understanding anxiety-related disorders. The reduction in anxiety that follows from avoidance behavior (staying away from the thing that the survivor thinks will make them think about the trauma) serves as a negative reinforcer, while preventing extinction of conditioned responses.

Orval Hobart Mowrer (1907–1982) is known for articulating the complementary relationship between classical and operant conditioning in his *two-factor theory* (Mowrer, 1960; Mowrer & Suter, 1950). According to Mowrer's theory, pathological fear develops via classical conditioning and is maintained via operant conditioning. In the application of Mowrer's theory to the treatment of anxiety-related disorders (Dollard & Muiller, 1950), classical conditioning explains the origins of the posttraumatic response. The stimuli that were originally paired with the traumatic event elicit the emotional, physiological, cognitive, and behavioral responses at subsequent presentations. Examples of specific stimuli that could elicit classically conditioned responses in an individual with combat-related PTSD could include the sound of fireworks or a car backfiring, smells of garbage, seeing sandy landscapes, or watching news or movies related to combat. Traumatic reactions can spread to stimuli less clearly related to the traumatic event through the process of generalization. Operant conditioning maintains the traumatic reactions through negative reinforcement of avoidance behavior. Examples of avoidance include explicitly staying away from crowded or noisy places, turning off news updates that may relate to war, not discussing the traumatic event, and isolating oneself in the home. Avoidance, in turn, prevents extinction, which is the process by which the individual learns that the conditioned stimuli no longer signal threat.

An early application of learning theory to the treatment of anxiety-related disorders was developed in 1954 by Joseph Wolpe (1915–1997), who believed that anxiety disorders could be treated through *reciprocal inhibition*, wherein patients are exposed to conditioned stimuli while engaging in deep muscle relaxation, which is incompatible with anxiety. Once the patient could remain in a relaxed state in the presence of the conditioned stimuli, they would be exposed to the next stimulus on their hierarchy of anxiety-provoking stimuli/situations. Later studies showed that relaxation was not necessary for extinction of the fear response to occur. In addition, the hierarchical approach was not necessary, because *flooding*, wherein the patient confronts the most anxiety-provoking stimuli/situation for an extended period, was also shown to be efficacious.

Keane et al. (1985) applied Mowrer's theory to understand the symptoms observed in Vietnam War veterans. They proposed that fear responding may be conditioned to a wide range of stimuli that are present during life-threatening war experiences. Through the process of stimulus generalization and higher order conditioning, stimuli not present during war experiences may also come to evoke distress responses. To explain why reexperiencing symptoms of PTSD does not extinguish the distress response, they proposed that these spontaneous exposures are incomplete, in that they do not include all relevant stimuli and are of too short a duration for extinction learning to occur. They further proposed that trauma memories may be incomplete because of efforts to avoid the intense distress that can arise when thinking about the event, efforts to avoid discussing the emotional impact of the trauma (they considered this particularly true for men due to gender socialization), and the discrepancy between the mood state during the trauma versus recall, which can hinder recall.

Applying the above conceptualization to the treatment of PTSD, Keane et al. (1985) suggested that extinction learning may be enhanced by providing more cues about the traumatic event and confronting the memory for a prolonged period of time. Foa et al. (1989) proposed that distress during the memory confrontation may enhance recall by reducing the discrepancy in mood between the trauma and the recall state.

Mowrer's theory was also used by Becker et al. (1984) and by Kilpatrick et al. (1985) to explain the aversion to sexual activities following sexual assault or rape. These researchers proposed that all the stimuli present during a sexual assault are classically conditioned by their pairing with the unconditioned stimulus of the assault. Through generalization and higher order conditioning, a wide range of intimate activities also come to evoke distress. Kilpatrick et al. further suggested that words associated with the trauma may also be conditioned to evoke distress. Efforts to inhibit sexual feelings and avoid intimate or sexual activity not only are relied upon to minimize distress but also serve to prevent extinction learning.

Keane and Barlow (2002) proposed an etiological model for anxiety-related disorders in which a biological vulnerability to experience negative affect and a psychological vulnerability to a diminished sense of control and anxiety apprehension together increased one's risk for developing anxiety-related disorders. Traumatic experiences are considered "true alarms," in that they are actually threatening, whereas conditioned stimuli are considered "false alarms." The preexisting vulnerabilities determine the probability that a traumatic experience will trigger a true alarm. Subsequent exposure to conditioned stimuli triggers false alarms, leading to anxious apprehension (e.g., hypervigilance) and avoidance behavior.

Mowrer's parsimonious and influential theory is useful for explaining many key features related to PTSD psychopathology, including the development of fear responding following trauma, the generalization of such responding to safe stimuli, the development of avoidance behaviors, and how avoidance prevents recovery. It is less clear how the development of reexperiencing symptoms of PTSD (intrusive thoughts and memories) is explained by conditioning processes.

SCHEMA THEORIES

Cognitive theory and science grew rapidly in the 1960s and 1970s, in part as a reaction to strict behaviorism, which viewed cognition and other nonobservable events as having no place in the field of psychology. One of the theoretical contributions of this work that was later applied to PTSD was the notion of a *cognitive schema*. In 1962, Jean Piaget (1896–1980) developed the idea that information congruent with existing mental frameworks or schemas is readily assimilated, whereas information that is discrepant with existing schemas requires that the schema be altered to accommodate the new information. Schemas help people understand their world, interpret new information, and guide decisions that help us navigate the environment. The notion of schemas or core assumptions and beliefs guiding the interpretation of new information has been influential in PTSD conceptualizations. Incorporating ideas from psychoanalytic theory and information processing, Horowitz (1986) proposed that recovery from trauma requires repetition of the trauma-related information with existing inner schemas or models until the two agree, referred to as the *completion tendency*. This repetition of trauma-related information is manifest in PTSD reexperiencing symptoms. In PTSD, the completion tendency is countered by the tendency to avoid distress-provoking thoughts and images, which prevents resolution of the discrepancy between trauma-related information and inner models.

Drawing on theory from social and personality psychology, Janoff-Bulman (1989) developed the *shattered assumptions theory*, another influential schema theory, based on the notion that people assume the world is generally benevolent and meaningful and that the self is intrinsically worthy. The experience of trauma disrupts these core assumptions and can drastically alter the way people view the world, themselves, and others. As a result of this disruption, the survivor must either assimilate the traumatic experience into their existing core assumption (e.g., by blaming oneself for the trauma and thereby protecting the belief in a just world) or change their core assumption to accommodate the traumatic experience (e.g., the world is not always benevolent). McCann and Pearlman (1990) proposed several fundamental psychological needs relevant to trauma survivors, including safety, trust, power, esteem, and intimacy. Similar to Janoff-Bulman, they proposed that the experience of a traumatic event disrupts the schemas related to these psychological needs, and that recovery from trauma should involve helping patients to accommodate their schemas with the new trauma-related information. McCann et al. (1988) demonstrated that beliefs about one's safety, trust of oneself and others, power and control, esteem, and intimacy can be particularly susceptible to disruptions after exposure to a traumatic event. They proposed that traumatic events may not always disrupt existing schemas but may instead reinforce preexisting negative schemas related to the self, others, and the world.

Building upon Piaget's work (1962) on assimilation and accommodation, Resick and Schnicke (1993) proposed that symptoms of posttraumatic stress can develop when trauma-relevant information is assimilated into existing schemas' belief structures (e.g., "the trauma happened because I was not careful"). Self-blame and hindsight biases are examples of strategies to assimilate trauma-relevant information without altering beliefs about the world being benevolent, just, and safe. In cases where patients hold negative schemas, trauma-relevant information may be easily assimilated, reinforcing the preexisting negative beliefs. Resick and Schnicke also proposed that patients may overaccommodate their schemas when processing trauma-relevant information (e.g., "no place is ever safe"). *Cognitive processing therapy* (CPT), an evidence-based treatment for PTSD, was designed to help patients shift their beliefs to appropriately accommodate trauma-relevant information (e.g., the world is generally safe). Because disruptions in schemas can keep trauma survivors "stuck" in their symptomology, CPT seeks to identify and challenge "stuck points" or inaccurate patterns of thinking. CPT therapists work to identify assimilated and overaccommodated stuck points to help patients shift their thinking toward a balanced and accurate perspective about the event (e.g., "Sometimes bad things happen even when one is generally careful. The trauma was not my fault.").

COGNITIVE THEORIES

A foundational assumption of cognitive theory as proposed by Aaron Beck et al. (Beck, 2009; Beck et al., 1979; Ellis, 1977) is that it is one's interpretation of an event, rather than the event itself, that gives rise to emotional reaction. The clinical application of this notion is that emotional reactions can be managed by shifting one's interpretation of events. One's interpretation of an event is evident by examining one's thoughts, which are often habitual and unnoticed (i.e., "automatic thoughts") and relate to emotional reactions in predictable ways. When automatic thoughts are distorted or dysfunctional, they can cause emotional reactions that are intensely negative or prolonged. Thus, the clinical application of this theory is to help patients attend to, challenge, and develop more accurate and helpful thoughts. Beck's cognitive theory did not focus on PTSD, other than to propose that unsafe stimuli were incorrectly interpreted as dangerous, and that a lack of self-confidence in managing stressful experiences may maintain PTSD symptoms.

Ehlers and Clark (2000) proposed a cognitive model of PTSD based in part on Beck's cognitive theory and influenced by emotional processing theory (EPT). According to this model, there are two key processes that interact to promote the development and maintenance of PTSD. The first is the patient's beliefs or appraisals of the traumatic event, or of the event's consequences, or both: specifically, beliefs about external threat (e.g., "the world is dangerous") and internal threat (e.g., "I'm incompetent") about what happened during or after the traumatic event. The second key process is the fragmented nature of the traumatic memory that does not incorporate other autobiographical memories that, during recall, feels as though it is happening in the present, giving rise to current threat appraisals. As a result of these threat appraisals, recall of the trauma memory is biased, such that trauma-relevant information that is consistent with the appraisals is retrieved selectively. In contrast, information that is inconsistent with the threat-related core beliefs is ignored, preventing opportunities to shift these perceptions. In this model, avoidance behavior is viewed as the consequence of ongoing threat appraisals (rather than a contributing cause, as in EPT), and therefore cognitive therapy based on this model focuses on correcting the core beliefs and assumptions thought to underlie PTSD symptomatology.

EMOTIONAL PROCESSING THEORY

EPT, developed by Foa and Kozak (1985, 1986), is a transdiagnostic theory that has informed the conceptualization of the development, maintenance, and recovery from anxiety-related disorders, including PTSD. Because EPT is the theoretical foundation for prolonged exposure (PE), this theory is described in greater detail relative to other theories.

Fear Structures

EPT was heavily influenced by the early learning theories described above and by P. J. Lang's (1977, 1979) *bioinformational theory of fear*. According to Lang, fear is represented in memory in cognitive structures comprised of stimulus, response, and meaning elements that function as a "blueprint" for avoiding or escaping danger. For example, a fear structure may include stimulus elements, such as a gun, that would connect with behavioral and physiological response elements, such as heart racing, running away, or hiding. These elements would also connect with meaning elements, such as "I might be killed." When stimuli in the environment are similar to any of the elements of the fear structure, activation spreads throughout the entire network. Thus, inputs matching any one part of the structure activate the entire structure.

An important contribution of EPT is that it distinguishes between normal and pathological fear structures. Pathological fear structures are distinct from normal fear structures in that the different elements do not accurately represent reality. When confronted by a realistically dangerous situation, such as seeing an oncoming car speeding toward you as you cross the street, activating a fear structure elicits an adaptive behavior (e.g., running toward the sidewalk) to keep you safe. However, the fear structure is considered pathological when the fear structure becomes activated by stimuli or responses that are not truly dangerous. Foa and Kozak (1986) proposed that specific pathological fear structures underlie anxiety-related disorders.

Foa and Rothbaum (1998) proposed that the traumatic memory associated with PTSD can be considered a specific pathological fear structure that includes exaggerated or erroneous connections between stimuli and responses that were present at the time of the trauma and their meaning, as well as pathological meaning elements. For example, the fear structure of an individual with combat-related PTSD may include *representations of stimuli*, such as roadside garbage (which hides improvised explosive devices in garrisons); *representations of responses*, such as increased sweating and muscle tension; and *representations of the meaning* assigned to the stimuli, such as "roadside garbage is dangerous" and "increased sweating means I'm afraid." While a survivor of an improvised explosive device blast during war may accurately associate seeing trash during combat with danger, outside of a war zone, garbage on the side of the road is not dangerous. Similarly, the fear structure of someone who was sexually assaulted at a music concert may include representations of stimuli, such as crowds of people; responses, such as freezing; and meanings, such as "crowds are dangerous." Both trauma survivors may have pathological meaning elements in their fear structures, such as "I should have prevented the trauma."

EPT postulates that disrupted perceptual processing at the time of the trauma can cause trauma memories to be more disorganized and fragmented, which in turn enhances the potential for erroneous associations. According to EPT, the fear structures that underlie PTSD are also characterized by the large number of stimulus representations in the network, such that a wide range of inputs may trigger activation of the fear network. PTSD fear structures are also characterized by representations of one's responses during and after the trauma and are associated with the meaning of self-incompetence (e.g., "I'm incompetent because I was afraid" or "I'm a weak person because I froze"). These erroneous perceptions promote avoidance of trauma-related thoughts, images, and situations, which prevents emotional processing and thereby maintains PTSD symptoms.

Natural Recovery Versus Development of PTSD

Following the experience of a traumatic event, most individuals experience symptoms that overlap with those of PTSD, including reexperiencing the event in response to reminders, hyperarousal, and avoidance of trauma-related stimuli (Breslau et al., 2005). For most individuals, these symptoms decrease over the weeks and months that follow. However, for a significant minority of individuals, the symptoms do not ameliorate, leading to the development of PTSD.

A unique strength of EPT is that it employs the same mechanisms to explain both natural and therapeutic recovery (Cahill & Foa, 2007). Specifically, after a traumatic event, survivors often view the world as extremely dangerous and themselves as unable to cope with stress. These perceptions reflect a fear structure that includes excessive stimulus elements that, although realistically safe, were associated with a meaning of danger during the trauma as well as with responses that, while adaptive at the time of the trauma, are associated with the meaning of incompetence. Natural recovery following a traumatic event occurs when the fear structure is repeatedly activated in the absence of feared outcomes. For most survivors, the pathological elements are corrected through engagement in daily activities that disconfirm them. As such, those who (a) allow themselves to think about the trauma, (b) talk about it with supportive others, (c) engage with trauma-related emotions, and (d) approach situations and stimuli that are reminders of the trauma without avoiding or escaping would be expected to naturally recover from a traumatic event. In contrast, individuals who (a) avoid thinking and talking about the traumatic memory, (b) suppress or distract from trauma-related emotions, and (c) do not resume their pretrauma daily functioning but instead (d) alter their behavior to avoid trauma reminders do not have the opportunity to incorporate disconfirming information. Risk for developing PTSD increases when the pathological elements of the fear structure are maintained rather than disconfirmed. Thus, avoidance serves as a critical factor in the development and maintenance of PTSD.

EPT also emphasizes cognitive factors, such as negative trauma-related beliefs related to development, maintenance, and recovery from PTSD. Trauma-related beliefs are inflexible, inaccurate perceptions of the self, the world, and others, such as viewing the world as extremely dangerous, oneself as incapable of coping with symptoms, and all others as being untrustworthy (Foa, Huppert, & Cahill, 2006). These beliefs may develop as a result of the traumatic event or they may exist previously and be strengthened by the traumatic event. EPT proposes that negative trauma-related beliefs also maintain PTSD by promoting avoidance (Foa, Huppert, & Cahill, 2006; Foa & Kozak, 1986).

Effective Psychological Treatment

According to EPT, effective psychological treatments for anxiety-related disorders, such as *exposure therapy*, work by promoting emotional processing, which involves modification of the pathological elements of the underlying fear structure. Specifically, there are two necessary conditions for modification of a fear structure. The first is that the fear structure must be activated so that it is available for modification. By analogy, a Word document must be opened in order to revise the content. Second, information that is incompatible with the pathological elements of the fear structure must be made available and integrated into the fear structure. This allows the pathological elements of the fear structure to be modified with more realistic elements that reflect the current context of life rather than the trauma context.

Exposure therapy is an effective approach to achieving these two conditions. Approaching anxiety-provoking but safe stimuli is likely to activate the pathological fear structure while also providing corrective information about the probability and cost of feared consequences (i.e., because feared outcomes do not occur). Thus, effective treatment for PTSD involves resuming avoided daily activities and engaging with the traumatic memory in order to disconfirm the pathological elements of the fear structure. Systematic repeated confrontation with traumatic memories (*imaginal exposure*) and avoided trauma-related situations (*in vivo exposure*) are an effective means of presenting patients with information that disconfirms the pathological elements of their fear structure, thereby facilitating recovery from PTSD. EPT's focus on incorporating disconfirming information is consistent with Rescorla and Wagner's (1972) mathematical model of classical conditioning, which proposed that extinction learning resulted from the discrepancy between what is expected to occur and what actually occurs. According to the Rescorla-Wagner mathematical model, this learning then modified future threat expectancies, which are like the meaning elements described in EPT.

Also influenced by modern learning theory that views extinction as the process of generating new nonfear associations (Bouton & Swartzentruber, 1991), Foa and McNally (1996) proposed that exposure therapy does not modify existing pathological fear structure but, instead, promotes the development of a new competing structure that does not include the same pathological associations among stimulus, response, and meaning representations. The pathological fear structure and the new realistic structure contain overlapping elements. As a result of this overlap, either may be activated by the same stimuli and responses. When therapy has been successful, the new structure is more easily activated when shared elements are present. In contrast, relapse occurs when the old, pathological fear structure is activated instead.

EPT as Applied to PE

According to EPT, effective psychological recovery from PTSD requires the activation of the fear structure and the presence of disconfirming information (i.e., lack of feared outcomes). The latter is easily achieved by selecting exposures to safe situations that are trauma reminders (or memories of the trauma, which are always safe). Activating the fear structure may require fine-tuning; both too little activation (underengagement) and too much activation (overengagement) may limit treatment efficacy. Underengagement occurs when the fear structure underlying PTSD is insufficiently activated. This is problematic because it prevents successful modification of the pathological fear structure. Underengagement may be observed in either in vivo or imaginal exposure. During imaginal exposure, underengagement may be suspected when the patient recounts the traumatic event in a detached or unemotional manner; excludes details about the event, particularly those related to thoughts and feelings that occurred; speaks with a flat or completely neutral appearance; and reports low levels of subjective distress.

Clinical strategies to increase patient engagement with the trauma memory, for the purpose of attaining optimal fear activation, include reminding the patient of the rationale for PE, inviting the patient to close their eyes, speak in the present tense, and include details about their thoughts, feelings, and actions, and probing for such details during the imaginal exposure. If underengagement continues, it can also help to role-play imaginal exposure using a non-traumatic-event example, thus modeling the level of detail requested and use of present tense.

The flip side of underengagement is overengagement. EPT asserts that they both function in the same way: to prevent processing of information that disconfirms the pathological elements in the fear structure. Overengagement occurs when the fear structure is too activated, such that it overwhelms the patient and prevents them from attending to the presence of disconfirming information. Like underengagement, overengagement can also occur during in vivo or imaginal exposure. During imaginal exposure, overengagement may be likely if the patient "acts out" part of the trauma memory with their gestures or by jumping in their seat. Excessive crying and high-reported subjective distress are also signs of overengagement. Imaginal exposure can be easily modified to prevent overengagement. In addition to reminding the patient of the rationale, the patient may be invited to use the past tense, open their eyes, limit details during the recounting, write and read the narrative of the trauma memory, and/or practice grounding techniques concurrently. Use of such techniques should be faded over the course of treatment as tolerated. Although strong affect is expected with effective PE, overengagement is much less common than underengagement, likely because patients with PTSD have learned to avoid trauma-related memories and feelings as a means of coping with their symptoms in the short term, making this avoidance habitual. As a result, most PE therapists end up working more often on ways to increase engagement rather than to reduce engagement.

As the fear structure is modified via repeated exposure to trauma memories and trauma-related situations and stimuli, the strength of the new realistic associations takes precedence over the erroneous associations, and excessive responding should therefore diminish. According to EPT, this process of extinction learning should be evidenced by a reduction in fear responding over time. When extinction is not evident over successive exposure sessions, several procedural issues may need to be remedied. First, it is important that the patient remain in the in vivo situations and engaged in the imaginal exposure for a long enough duration for disconfirmation to occur. If the patient escapes the situation too early, this may reinforce the idea that it was in fact dangerous. Second, it is important to ensure that the patient is not engaging in subtle avoidance or in safety behaviors that may interfere with extinction. If safety behaviors go unchecked, the patient may attribute the lack of feared outcomes to the safety behavior rather than the safety of the situation. Finally, it is important that the exposure be repeated, as many times as needed, to achieve extinction. Once extinction in the same context is achieved, the exposure may be attempted in different contexts for the purpose of promoting generalization.

Indicators of Emotional Processing

Emotional processing is described by Foa and Kozak (1986) as a multistep process that involves activation of the fear structure, also called *emotional engagement*, and the incorporation of disconfirming evidence that is incompatible with the erroneous elements of the pathological fear structure. Repeated exposures to trauma reminders in daily life (i.e., in vivo exposure) and to trauma memories (i.e., imaginal exposure) promote fear extinction. Foa and Kozak (1986) proposed three indicators of successful emotional processing. The first indicator, *activation of the fear structure*, which is prerequisite for modification of the pathological elements to occur, is indicated by both subjective and objective measures of anxious arousal. The second indicator is *within-session extinction* (WSE), or the reduction of anxiety within a treatment session. The final indicator is *between-session extinction* (BSE), meaning the reduction in peak anxiety across treatment sessions. Evidence for the relevance of each of these processes to therapeutic recovery will be evaluated in turn in Chapter 3 (see also A. A. Cooper, Clifton, & Feeny, 2017; Craske et al., 2008, for reviews of this evidence).

Mechanisms of Emotional Processing

EPT proposes that emotional activation, WSE, and BSE are indicators that emotional processing is taking place. There has been some confusion about this issue in the field, but these indicators were not proposed as mechanisms that drive emotional processing but instead indicators that processing is happening. Separate from the above indicators, EPT proposed potential mechanisms of therapeutic recovery during exposure therapy (Foa, Hembree, et al., 2019; Foa & Kozak, 1986; Foa & McLean, 2016; S. A. M. Rauch & Foa, 2006). These include the organization and elaboration of the trauma narrative and changes in negative trauma-related cognitions.

Organization of the Trauma Memory

As described by Foa and Riggs (1993) and Ehlers and Clark (2000), memories of traumatic events are often characterized by disorganization and fragmentation, particularly for those with PTSD. Consistent with this observation, Amir et al. (1998) found that the PTSD severity was positively correlated with the degree to which trauma narratives of rape survivors were organized and articulated. Several subsequent studies (Buck et al., 2006; Halligan et al., 2003; Jones et al., 2007; Murray et al., 2002), but not all (Gray & Lombardo, 2001), have found a significant relationship between trauma narrative organization and PTSD status (O'Kearney & Perrott, 2006). Jaeger et al. (2014) found that the content of trauma narratives (more positive and negative emotion words, higher cognitive process, and less self-focus) but not the structure of the narratives (e.g., fragmentation, disorganization) was associated with lower PTSD symptoms.

EPT proposes that one of the mechanisms of therapeutic recovery from PTSD is the organization and elaboration of the trauma memory narrative (Foa & Jaycox, 1999). According to EPT, the repeated revisiting and articulation of the trauma memory during imaginal exposure helps to reorganize and elaborate the trauma narrative, thereby driving emotional processing and recovery. Two small studies (*Ns* < 20) examined this tenant of EPT using a qualitative coding system. Foa, Molnar, and Cashman (1995) found that trauma narratives at the end of PE were longer and more organized than trauma narratives at the beginning of PE and that the degree of reduction in fragmentation and increase in organization across treatment was associated with PTSD symptom reduction. Using a similar design, van Minnen et al. (2002) also found an increase in organization and inclusion of thoughts and feelings in trauma narratives from pre- to posttreatment, and that these changes were greater among those classified as improved.

Consistent with EPT, these studies found that some measures of organization, including planning and decision making (Foa, Molnar, & Cashman, 1995), and organized thoughts (van Minnen et al., 2002) were associated with improvement in PTSD symptoms across PE. Inconsistent with EPT, the degree of memory fragmentation either did not change during PE (Foa, Molnar, & Cashman, 1995) or was not greater among those classified as improved (van Minnen et al., 2002). Null findings for a relationship between memory fragmentation and PTSD symptom improvement were also found in subsequent larger studies (Kindt et al., 2007; Moulds & Bryant, 2005). These inconsistencies may be due to the use of subjective coding protocols and small sample sizes. However, in a recent and large PTSD trial that used self-report, rater coding, and objective coding of trauma memory narrative content, Bedard-Gilligan et al. (2017) found that, although sensory components of the narrative increased during PE, there were no consistent differences in fragmentation from pre- to posttreatment between responders and nonresponders. Thus, contrary to EPT, it may be that trauma memory organization is not a mechanism of therapeutic recovery during PE.

Changes in Negative Trauma-Related Cognitions

Early iterations of EPT (Foa & Kozak, 1986) focused on the modification of meaning and stimulus associations, such as the shift in viewing the trauma memory itself as dangerous, that occurred as the memory was repeatedly confronted in a safe therapeutic context. Such shifts were linked to exposure exercises that provided disconfirming evidence relevant to negative trauma-related beliefs. More recent descriptions of EPT (Foa & McLean, 2016) focused on the mechanistic role of shifts in negative trauma-related cognitions with less direct links to specific exposure techniques. Importantly, EPT proposes that there are interactions among various processes, such that the experience of WSE and BSE provides disconfirming evidence (e.g., evidence that distress will persist indefinitely in the absence of avoidance or escape). These interactions can lead to changes in trauma-related cognitions. Indeed, this overlap is likely the cause of some confusion around the distinction between indicators and mechanisms of emotional processing.

Like the schema theories described earlier, EPT proposes that trauma can significantly impact survivors' view of themselves, others, and the world. Specifically, EPT proposes that PTSD is maintained, in part, by negative trauma-related cognitions or perceptions that the world is entirely dangerous, that others are entirely untrustworthy, and that the self is entirely incompetent (Foa & Riggs, 1993). Accordingly, therapeutic recovery from PTSD involves correcting these negative trauma-related cognitions.

In contrast to the tenets of EPT reviewed above, the evidence supporting change in negative trauma-related cognitions (e.g., "I'm incompetent," "The world is completely dangerous," "No one can be trusted"), typically measured by the Posttraumatic Cognitions Inventory (PTCI; Foa, Ehlers, et al., 1999) as a potential mechanism of change during PE, is quite strong. Providing initial indirect evidence for the role of negative trauma-related cognitions, Foa and Rauch (2004) reported that negative cognitions reduced over the course of PE and that these reductions were significantly correlated with improvements in PTSD among women assault survivors receiving PE. Using a different measure, Paunovic and Öst (2001) found similar results among torture survivors with PTSD receiving PE. Overall pre- to posttreatment changes in negative trauma-related cognitions have been found to correlate with overall PTSD symptom reduction (Nacasch et al., 2015). Moreover, changes in trauma-related cognitions have also been shown to predict subsequent changes in PTSD symptoms during exposure therapy (Øktedalen et al., 2015).

Subsequent mediation studies offered more direct evidence for a potential mechanistic role of negative cognitions. Zalta et al. (2014) found that reductions in negative trauma-related cognitions temporally preceded decreases in PTSD symptoms in a trial of PE among women with assault-related PTSD, whereas evidence for the reverse relationship (i.e., PTSD change preceding negative cognition change) was not found. This finding was replicated in a subsequent study of civilians with mixed trauma using a similar analytic approach (Kumpula et al., 2017). Change in negative trauma-related cognitions was found to mediate change in PTSD symptoms in a sample of civilians with comorbid mixed-trauma-related PTSD and alcohol dependence receiving PE (McLean, Su, & Foa, 2015). Mediation was also observed among adolescents with sexual assault–related PTSD receiving PE, and, contrary to hypothesis, among those receiving supportive counseling as well, albeit to a lesser degree (McLean, Yea, et al., 2015). Similar findings were observed by A. A. Cooper, Zoellner, et al. (2017), who found that changes in trauma-related cognitions temporally preceded changes in PTSD among those receiving PE or sertraline, although this effect was much stronger in PE ($d = 0.93$) than sertraline ($d = 0.35$). Two studies found that change in negative trauma-related cognitions mediates change in PTSD symptoms among those receiving PE and those receiving present-centered therapy, a non-trauma-focused treatment (McLean et al., 2019; S. A. M. Rauch, King, et al., 2015). These latter findings suggested that changes in negative cognitions may mediate reductions in PTSD symptoms across treatment types (see also Ehlers et al., 2003) rather than in PE, trauma-focused therapy, or even psychotherapy specifically. A limitation of this literature is that, to date, only one study has tested an alternate mediator of PTSD change during PE, finding preliminary evidence that negative trauma-related cognitions may not be the most important mediator of change (McLean et al., 2019). More research on alternate candidate mediators of change will help determine the specificity of trauma-related cognitions as mediators of therapeutic recovery.

INHIBITORY LEARNING THEORY

Inhibitory learning theory (Craske et al., 2008, 2014) is a transdiagnostic model based on classic learning paradigms showing that return of fear is common following extinction (Bouton, 1993). PTSD is conceptualized as resulting from the pairing of the traumatic experience (unconditioned stimulus [US]) with a variety of sensory and contextual information (neutral stimulus), such that the previously neutral stimuli come to activate the trauma memory (conditioned stimulus [CS]; Bouton, 1993). After extinction or exposure therapy, the CS possesses two meanings: the original excitatory meaning (CS-US) and the new inhibitory meaning (CS-noUS). Through repeated exposure to the CS in the absence of feared outcomes and in a variety of contexts, the competing association (CS-noUS) becomes more likely to be activated in response to CS than the original CS-US association. However, the original association is never fully erased and is subject to spontaneous recovery following the passage of time (Craske & Mystkowski, 2006; Craske & Rachman, 1987); renewal of conditional fear, when a CS is presented in a context where exposure had not previously occurred (Culver et al., 2011; Mystkowski et al., 2002, 2003, 2006); reinstatement of conditional fear when unpaired US presentations occur (Hermans et al., 2005; Rescorla & Heth, 1975; Van Damme et al., 2006); and rapid reacquisition when the CS-US pairing is repeated (e.g., retraumatization).

The idea of the competing associations in inhibitory learning is like EPT's notion of a competing fear/emotion network, with the new safety association being strengthened through exposures. An additional similarity between the two theories is the focus on emotional engagement during exposure (e.g., Culver et al., 2012). A central point of divergence is that, whereas EPT views the reduction of distress during treatment as an indicator of therapeutic change and as a potential source of disconfirming evidence that shifts negative trauma-related cognitions, inhibitory learning theory considers the reduction in distress as unrelated to the strengthening of the competing inhibitory association (Craske et al., 2014) and changes in trauma-related beliefs are not considered central to therapeutic recovery (Graham & Milad, 2011). Inhibitory learning theory draws a distinction between fear expression during exposure and therapeutic learning. Distress may not decline while inhibitory learning occurs, and it is the learning, not performance during the exposure, that is critical to outcomes. Instead of fear reduction, inhibitory learning theory emphasizes fear tolerance during exposure as an adaptive emotion regulation strategy. On the basis of evidence that individuals with anxiety-related disorders have deficits in the mechanisms thought to be central to extinction learning, inhibitory learning models have focused on identifying and testing ways to optimize inhibitory learning during exposure as a means of improving exposure outcomes and addressing the deficits among those with anxiety-related disorders. Strategies aim to strengthen inhibitory learning such that the probability of spontaneous recovery, renewal, reinstatement, and reacquisition decreases as the retrieval strength of the CS-noUS association increases (Craske et al., 2014, 2018; Weisman & Rodebaugh, 2018). The goal is to develop new, nonthreat associations and to enhance the accessibility and retrievability of these associations over time and a wide variety of contexts.

For the remainder of this book, we draw upon these theories as we explore the application of neuroscience findings to the practice of PE. Wherever possible, we present the findings from neuroscience as they do or do not conform to these theorized mechanisms of change in order to assist PE providers in applying the latest research to improve their practice of PE on the individual patient level.

2 WHAT IS PROLONGED EXPOSURE THERAPY?

Exposure therapy is a type of cognitive behavioral therapy (CBT) designed to reduce pathological anxiety and related emotions by helping patients approach relatively safe but distress-provoking thoughts, memories, situations, and stimuli, with the goal of reducing unhelpful emotional reactions to those stimuli. Prolonged exposure (PE) is one specific and highly studied protocol for providing exposure therapy for posttraumatic stress disorder (PTSD). Exposure therapy originated from theory-driven research on learning and behavior. It was the first psychological treatment for which the procedures were described in detail, allowing replication among researchers and application among therapists treating patients with anxiety-related disorders. Beginning in the 1960s and continuing to date, exposure therapies have been extensively developed, studied, and refined. There are several variants of exposure therapy, including *imaginal exposure, in vivo exposure, systematic desensitization*, and *interoceptive exposure*. The selection of the type of exposure is determined by the characteristics of a given disorder. Often, several types of exposure are used concurrently in exposure therapy programs for specific disorders, such as PTSD, panic disorder, or social anxiety disorder.

https://doi.org/10.1037/0000242-002
Retraining the Brain: Applied Neuroscience in Exposure Therapy for PTSD,
by S. A. M. Rauch and C. P. McLean

DEVELOPMENT OF PROLONGED EXPOSURE THERAPY

PE therapy is a specific manualized exposure therapy program for PTSD. It was developed in the 1980s, following the addition of PTSD in the third edition of the *Diagnostic and Statistical Manual of Mental Disorders* (*DSM-III*; American Psychiatric Association, 1987), and has been studied extensively, with revised criteria put forward in 2013 with *DSM-5* (American Psychiatric Association, 2013). Prior to 1980, PTSD was not formally recognized and there was little understanding of how best to treat the disorder. However, evidence for the efficacy of exposure therapy for anxiety-related conditions was well documented by this time, and some therapists were having success applying exposure therapy to treat trauma survivors who were haunted by trauma memories. It was in this context that Foa et al. (2007) developed the first PE program. The first treatment manual was published in 2007, and a revised and updated version was published in 2019 (Foa, Hembree, et al., 2019). The key components of PE are (a) psychoeducation about the nature of trauma, what maintains trauma reactions, and how PE reduces these reactions; (b) in vivo exposure to trauma reminders; and (c) imaginal exposure to the memory of the traumatic event followed by processing of the imaginal and other exposures. While processing has a key role in PE that is discussed in detail in later chapters, it occurs within the context of exposures and not as an independent component and, as such, they are combined into one component.

PE is based on *emotional processing theory* (EPT; Foa & Kozak, 1986), which conceptualizes PTSD as a failure to process the trauma memory due to avoidance of thoughts and situations related to the trauma. Avoidance then prevents the trauma survivor from learning that those thoughts and situations are not dangerous (or not as dangerous as they feel). Further, for many trauma survivors, each time they avoid trauma-related stimuli they believe they are confirming that they cannot handle thinking about the memory, facing situations associated with the memory, and negative affect more generally. Avoidance maintains and even feeds individuals' unhelpful negative perceptions about themselves and the world and prevents emotional processing from occurring. Accordingly, the goal of PE is to promote emotional processing through deliberately and systematically approaching trauma-related stimuli. In vivo exposure to trauma reminders in daily life and imaginal exposure to the trauma memory followed by discussion of the imaginal exposure experience and their thoughts about the self and world related to that experience (processing) are used concurrently during PE in order to disconfirm the unhelpful negative perceptions that underlie PTSD and help the survivor feel more able to handle the memory and negative affect more generally.

Most individuals who are exposed to a traumatic event experience some symptoms similar to PTSD, including reexperiencing the traumatic event in response to trauma reminders, hyperarousal, and avoidance of trauma-related stimuli (e.g., Breslau et al., 2005). For most trauma survivors, these symptoms ameliorate over time. When symptom reduction does not occur, PTSD develops. Applying EPT to PTSD, Foa and Cahill (2001) suggested that natural recovery following a trauma occurs when the emotion structure is repeatedly activated in the absence of feared consequences. Thus, individuals who think and talk about the traumatic event, engage with trauma-related feelings, and approach reminders of the trauma in daily life would be expected to recover from a traumatic event (see also Foa, Stein, & McFarlane, 2006). In contrast, individuals who avoid the traumatic memory and trauma-related stimuli develop PTSD, and their lives become smaller and smaller as their avoidance grows over time.

Foa and Rothbaum (1989) proposed that the traumatic memories associated with PTSD can be conceived as a specific pathological fear structure that includes erroneous associations among stimuli and responses and their meaning. Although these structures form normally for all of us following trauma, they are maintained over time through avoidance. Upon exposure to trauma, everything present during the trauma is included in an initial trauma structure. For example, for a combat soldier who experienced an attack on her convoy by a roadside improvised explosive device (IED), everything present at the time of the explosion is initially in the structure. Stimuli include the garbage, nighttime, hot weather, streets by the city market, and even the smell of sweat. Responses include her heart racing, increased respiration, and sweating. Meaning items include "I was afraid," "This experience and my reactions define me in some way," and "This was dangerous." Associations between these items may be helpful or unhelpful and realistic or unrealistic. Often these associations may change in their value with context. For instance, garbage by the road is not dangerous in the context of garbage day back home in Illinois. However, garbage by the road in Afghanistan can hide IEDs and is dangerous. In the acute aftermath of trauma, these associations are present and, as the trauma survivor reengages with life and the context where they reside, are modified to fit the new environment and overall risk.

When avoidance occurs instead of reengagement following trauma, then the structure and associations remain and may even strengthen and grow over time as the survivor becomes more convinced of the unhelpful associations, especially those related to their sense of incompetence and inability to handle negative affect. The fear structure of an individual with PTSD will include representations of stimuli, as well as response and meaning elements and their associations. According to S. A. M. Rauch and Foa (2006), the emotion structure underlying PTSD is characterized by a large number of stimulus representations that are erroneously associated with threat and that representations of the responses during the trauma and of PTSD symptoms are associated with the meaning of self-incompetence (e.g., "My reaction during the trauma and my PTSD symptoms mean that I am a weak person"). These erroneous perceptions drive additional avoidance of trauma-related thoughts, images, and situations, which prevents emotional processing and thereby maintains PTSD symptoms.

OVERVIEW OF TREATMENT

PE typically consists of eight to 15 individual 90-minute sessions, although recent findings suggest it is equally effective when delivered in 60-minute sessions (Foa et al., 2020; Nacasch et al., 2015). PE has been found effective when delivered in many ways. Although traditionally implemented in once- or twice-weekly sessions, it can also be delivered successfully in massed, daily sessions (Foa et al., 2018) and in a brief format delivered in primary care (Cigrang et al., 2017). PE has also been found effective when delivered via telehealth (Acierno et al., 2017; Yuen et al., 2015) and even through a therapist-supported online program (McLean et al., 2020).

In the first session, the therapist provides an overview of treatment and a rationale for PE and explains the procedures that will be used in the treatment and how they work to address the factors that maintain PTSD symptoms. The first session also involves an interview to collect information about the trauma, the patient's reactions to the trauma, and pre-trauma-stressful experiences. This interview concludes with a decision about which trauma to focus on during imaginal exposure. For patients who have experienced multiple traumas, this "index trauma" is selected by determining which trauma is currently causing the most distress and dysfunction. This event is often the one that is associated with the most frequent and upsetting reexperiencing symptoms. Depending on symptoms connected to additional traumas, the therapist may plan to focus exclusively on one trauma, as it seems to drive most of the PTSD-related symptoms, or may create a hierarchy of traumas, if there are a few that have unique meaning and specific connected symptoms. If multiple traumas are planned for exposure in the episode of care, typically no more than three would be planned, and the standard protocol is to begin with the most difficult and work down from there. This is based on the idea that generalization and reduction in PTSD symptoms as the patient works on the most difficult memory will generalize to the less difficult memory, often resulting in few or no remaining symptoms to address when the therapist and patient get to the second or third memory. Such generalization is not expected if the therapist and patient work up from the easiest memory. In addition to selecting the event, the therapist and patient agree upon the beginning and end points of the index trauma memory that will be used to structure the imaginal exposure. Finally, the first session also involves teaching patients a slow, diaphragmic breathing technique as a general stress reduction technique (not to be used during exposure) that they are encouraged to practice daily as homework. Additional homework includes reading a handout on the rationale for PE, tracking their slow breathing practice, and listening to the audio recording of the session one time.

The second session begins with reviewing homework and then moves to an in-depth discussion of common reactions to trauma. This discussion provides the patient with a framework for understanding their PTSD symptoms and associated problems and gives them the opportunity to share information about their experience of trauma. Next, the therapist introduces in vivo exposure and works with the patient to construct a hierarchy by listing and rank ordering previously avoided or anxiety-provoking situations related to the trauma, based on how distressed the patient would expect to be if they approached the situation. After creating the in vivo hierarchy, specific in vivo assignments are selected for homework. Patients typically practice two to three situations each week and move up the hierarchy as they conquer each item. Patients are asked to track their progress with in vivo exposure exercises for homework for the remainder of treatment. Continued breathing retraining and listening to the audio recording of the session one time are set homework exercises throughout treatment.

In the third session, after reviewing the homework, the therapist presents a rationale for imaginal exposure and then spends most of the session conducting imaginal exposure (at least 40 minute per session). Imaginal exposure involves asking the patient to revisit the memory of the trauma in their imagination and recount the event in detail aloud, typically with eyes closed and using the present tense. Imaginal exposure is followed by about 15 minutes of postexposure "processing" of thoughts and feelings related to the trauma with the aim of helping the patient see the trauma and their behaviors at the time of the trauma in the trauma context. This new view often results in modifications to the trauma structure that may include changes in the associations to reflect a more helpful perspective about the event itself and about the patient's behaviors and emotions during the trauma. Processing also includes a discussion of the patient's experiences during the imaginal exposure and focuses on the lessons learned from the experience. Specifically, the focus is on making the implicit learning explicit and pointing out the instances of approaching the trauma, instead of avoiding them, and the patient's successes (large and small) in approaching the trauma. Imaginal exposure is conducted in each subsequent session. In addition to the breathing practice, continued in vivo exposure, and listening to the entire session once, patients are instructed to listen to the recording of the imaginal exposure (recorded separately) each day as part of their weekly homework.

The remainder of treatment (Sessions 4 to up to 14) follows a standard agenda that begins with a review of the homework from the prior session. As treatment progresses, patients are encouraged to include greater detail about the index trauma and their reaction to it during the imaginal exposure and to focus more on the most distressing parts of the memory ("hot spots"). New homework exposure exercises are assigned at the end of the session. In the final treatment session, after homework is reviewed, the patient is asked to recount the full index trauma memory once (15–25 minutes). This imaginal exposure is followed by processing with an emphasis on how the experience of imaginal exposure has changed over the course of treatment. The therapist and patient also review progress, discuss the lessons learned, and plan for how the patient can maintain the gains made during treatment. The goal is for the patient to terminate treatment having successfully shifted their approach to managing PTSD symptoms from avoiding, which maintains anxiety, to approaching trauma reminders, which promotes recovery and mastery. They can then take their life back from PTSD.

Psychoeducation

Psychoeducation in PE involves explaining that PTSD symptoms are maintained by two factors. The first factor is avoidance of thoughts and images related to the trauma (i.e., cognitive avoidance) and avoidance of trauma reminders in daily life (i.e., behavioral avoidance). The therapist explains that, although avoidance is effective in reducing anxiety in the short term, it maintains PTSD symptoms in the long term by preventing opportunities to emotionally process the trauma memory. The second factor is the presence of unhelpful, distorted beliefs that have developed in the wake of the trauma. For example, many trauma survivors hold the belief that the world is extremely dangerous all or most of the time and that they are completely incompetent. The therapist then explains how PE alters these negative, distorted perceptions by providing opportunities to obtain corrective information that disconfirms these beliefs via experiential learning (i.e., exposure).

In addition to providing education about the rationale for PE, the therapist also provides education about common reactions to trauma. Reviewing common reactions can help the patient realize that their difficulties are recognized as PTSD symptoms, that the therapist is familiar with these symptoms, and that PE is geared toward alleviating these symptoms. The collaborative discussion about common reactions to trauma serves several aims. First, it provides an opportunity for the therapist to learn more about the patient's unique experience of PTSD symptoms and related problems. By explaining to the patient that these reactions are common and expected, the patient's experience is validated and normalized. Patients often find it helpful to understand that many of their seemingly disparate difficulties may in fact be related to PTSD, either directly or indirectly. Recognizing the interrelatedness of various symptoms can instill hope, in that reducing PTSD symptoms through PE may lead to an improvement in a variety of problem areas. Finally, the discussion of common reactions also provides an opportunity to learn about the patient's avoidance behaviors. Patients are not always aware of their avoidance patterns and may have difficulty generating a list of avoided situations for in vivo exposure. Patients may also be more willing to disclose avoidance in the context of the common reactions discussion than when generating an in vivo list that will be used to select homework assignments.

In Vivo Exposure

In vivo exposure refers to approaching places, people, and objects that the patient avoids because they remind them of the trauma and cause emotional distress (i.e., anxiety, shame, guilt) or because they feel unsafe since the trauma. In vivo exposures are designed to target PTSD patients' erroneous perceptions that safe situations are dangerous and should therefore be avoided; that their distress will continue indefinitely if they stay in the situation; and that they will not be able to tolerate the distress they experience. Consequently, in vivo exposure exercises involve approaching relatively safe situations that patients perceive to be dangerous (e.g., driving on highways for fear of an IED), as well as situations that they avoid because the situations are trauma reminders and cause high distress (e.g., watching news stories related to war). Thus, in vivo exposures are designed to achieve the two necessary conditions for emotional processing: activation of the trauma memory structure and disconfirmation of the expected disasters.

First, the therapist and patient collaboratively develop a list of safe or low-risk situations that the patient currently either avoids or endures with discomfort. The list should consider three types of situations: (a) situations that the patient perceives as dangerous (but are objectively safe or low risk) because the patient views the world as a dangerous place and has difficulty distinguishing between safe and unsafe situations, (b) situations and stimuli that are reminders of the trauma, and (c) situations or activities that the patient has lost interest in since the trauma (e.g., socializing, hobbies). For each situation on the list, the patient then assigns a *subjective units of distress* (SUDS) rating ranging from 0 to 100 as a means of rank ordering the situations based on how distressed they expect they would feel if they were to approach that situation now. A SUDS of 0 indicates no distress or anxiety at all, whereas a SUDS of 100 indicates the most distressed a person has ever been. A well-constructed hierarchy includes a range of items spanning from situations that generate moderate anxiety to those that generate the most anxiety a patient can imagine.

In vivo exposure is generally conducted in a stepwise fashion, beginning with situations that are moderately fear provoking before moving up the hierarchy to more challenging situations. This graduated approach helps patients build confidence and self-efficacy through early success experiences and is widely considered more palatable to patients than beginning with the most feared situations on the hierarchy. Importantly, in vivo exposure is only recommended for situations for which there is a relatively low probability of danger. Approaching objectively unsafe situations is neither appropriate nor therapeutic. For patients who live in more dangerous living conditions, this may include discussion of how others who live in that area would perceive the risk and what they might do to get their needs met within the lowest risk possible. For instance, for a patient who resides in a high-crime neighborhood, many of her neighbors would only walk to the grocery store with a companion and during daylight. For this patient to have a reasonable quality of life, she needs to be able to work within her current situation to get groceries for her family. Although we also discussed if and how to move to a safer area, ensuring that she could do the things she needed to do in her current situation was part of what helped to empower her and reduce her PTSD symptoms. The PE therapist does not ignore the fact that bad things can happen but tries to minimize the risk and support people to reach their goals.

The duration of exposure to the feared situation is considered an important factor in treating PTSD. The exposure must last long enough for corrective learning to occur (i.e., for the patient to associate the feared stimulus with safety and/or learn that they can tolerate the distress that they experience). Duration of 30 and 60 minutes appears to be sufficient for good outcomes (van Minnen & Foa, 2006), but the specific amount of time recommended will vary depending on the nature of the exposure. In general, it is recommended that the patient stay in the situation until their SUDS reduce by a significant amount, such as 50% or more. Although the reduction in SUDS that occurs within an exposure exercise is no longer considered critical for improvement (e.g., Foa, Huppert, & Cahill, 2006), it may be important for patients who hold erroneous beliefs about the consequences of anxiety (e.g., that it will be intolerable or will persist indefinitely).

Patients are instructed to begin doing in vivo exposures for homework between sessions beginning in Session 2. Each exposure situation on the hierarchy should be approached multiple times, with the goal of being able to enter the situation with minimal distress. In contrast to exposure therapy for other anxiety-related disorders, in vivo exposure in PE is conducted entirely as homework. There are several reasons for this. First, the situations that are typically feared and avoided by patients with PTSD are often difficult to access or simulate within a therapist's office. Second, conducting in vivo exposures independently for homework increases internal attribution of the patient's success experience. If a therapist is present, this internal attribution is less likely to occur. Third, exposures should occur wherever the patient's anxiety "lives" in order to promote generalization of extinction learning. PTSD does not live in the therapist's office.

When the patient is unable to initiate an in vivo exercise on their own, the therapist may suggest that the patient enlist the help of others, such as the patient's partner, friends, or family members. Including others can decrease the level of expected distress associated with an exposure exercise and is therefore a helpful strategy for modifying the difficulty of the in vivo assignment. Therapist assistance with in vivo exposures is warranted if the patient is persistently having difficulty completing assignments. In such cases, the therapist may accompany the patient when feasible to lend support and guidance. However, because therapist presence may serve as a "safety behavior" for the patient, it is essential for the patient to realize that they can complete in vivo exposure exercises and effectively manage their anxiety on their own. In any case, where someone else accompanies the patient in exposure, the goals would generally remain that this accompanied exposure is a step toward later moving to doing the in vivo exposure solo.

Safety behaviors refer to any behavior or mental actions used during exposure to reduce anxiety or prevent feared outcomes from occurring (e.g., standing near an exit; carrying a weapon; thinking, "If I pray when I do this, I'll be OK"). These behaviors can interfere with successful learning during exposure therapy because the patient attributes the absence of feared outcomes to having engaged in the safety behavior rather than to the fact that the situation was safe and that they could handle their distress. The availability of safety behaviors has been shown to be detrimental to exposure therapy among phobic samples (e.g., Freeman et al., 2007; McManus et al., 2008), whereas explicit instruction to withdraw safety behaviors has been shown to improve anxiety treatment outcomes (Salkovskis et al., 2007). Although, there is also evidence showing that some use of safety behaviors, particularly in the early stages of exposure therapy, may help patients with anxiety-related disorders engage in exposures (Hood et al., 2010; Milosevic & Radomsky, 2008). However, in the only study of safety behaviors and PTSD treatment to date, the reduction of safety behaviors during PE predicted greater improvement in PTSD severity (Goodson & Haeffel, 2018). The current PE protocol recommends assessing for safety behaviors and instructing patients not to use them.

In vivo exposure promotes therapeutic recovery by activating the emotional structure and correcting exaggerated probability estimates of harm. By intentionally approaching trauma reminders and remaining in the situation long enough to learn that feared outcomes do not occur and that the distress is tolerable, the pathological elements of the patient's trauma structure are disconfirmed. In vivo exposure provides the opportunity to test feared consequences and incorporate more realistic information through experiential learning. In vivo exposure also provides opportunities for extinction learning as patients learn that when they remain in the avoided situation for long enough, their distress decreases over time. Approaching and remaining in distressing trauma-related situations also prevents the negative reinforcement of avoidance and escape behaviors, which maintain PTSD. Successfully approaching feared situations can also help patients shift negative beliefs about themselves by promoting a sense of mastery and self-efficacy.

Imaginal Exposure

Imaginal exposure comprises a large part of the PE session. During imaginal exposure, the patient revisits the traumatic experience in their memory and verbally recounts the unfolding of events in detail. After providing a thorough rationale for the use of imaginal exposure in ameliorating PTSD symptoms, the therapist instructs the patient to close their eyes and describe aloud what happened during the trauma, while visualizing the event as vividly as possible. Patients are encouraged to include as much detail as possible, including information about the associated thoughts, feelings, and physical sensations they experienced during the trauma. Patients are also asked to close their eyes and use the present tense during the recounting as a means of promoting engagement with the memory. Imaginal exposure is continued for at least 40 minutes and includes multiple repetitions of the memory, as time permits, that begin and end at the points in the narrative that were agreed upon during Session 1. Once begun, imaginal exposure is typically conducted in each subsequent treatment session, as well as between sessions as homework by listening to an audio recording of the imaginal exposure daily.

Imaginal exposure activates the trauma structure and creates a powerful opportunity for new learning. Once the memory is activated it brings to the surface the unhelpful or unrealistic beliefs that maintain the symptoms of PTSD and allows for new insights into their beliefs about the self and the world. However, patients may have difficulty identifying and integrating disconfirming information that emerges from imaginal exposure on their own. Processing is conducted immediately after imaginal exposure in order to explore the trauma memory in its context and discuss how it relates to the patient's beliefs. The imaginal exposure can be thought of as providing a window into the trauma memory, and, once opened, there is an opportunity to reexamine everything connected to the trauma memory to determine whether it is accurate or inaccurate, helpful or unhelpful, and even whether it is something you want to continue to believe or whether your beliefs need to change as a result of further examination. Encouraging patients to elaborate on new insights and making insights explicit facilitate emotional processing and modification of the trauma structure underlying PTSD in a therapeutic direction.

There are several ways in which imaginal exposure is thought to help patients recover from PTSD. First, like in vivo exposure, repeatedly revisiting the trauma memory promotes extinction of conditioned distress reactions (i.e., extinction learning). This reduces the intensity of the distressing emotions that were associated with the trauma memory and helps to correct the patient's erroneous belief that recalling the trauma memory is dangerous or harmful (e.g., will cause the patient to "go crazy" or "lose control") or that their distress will last forever if they do not push the memory away. Revisiting and recounting the most distressing traumatic memory in imagination is designed to help the patient learn that engaging with the trauma memory does not result in harm and that they can tolerate the distress that the memory evokes. In turn, this learning alters negative perceptions about lacking self-efficacy and self-control.

Second, deliberately approaching the trauma memory prevents the negative reinforcement of avoidance. *Negative reinforcement* is the feeling of relief that people get when a perceived negative outcome is stopped, removed, or avoided. A standard example of negative reinforcement is when a child screams until they get a toy. For the parent, they are working to "remove" the negative outcome of the screaming. For a trauma survivor, pushing away trauma memories usually leads to an immediate decrease in distress that, although temporary, reinforces the avoidance behaviors that maintain PTSD. By approaching the trauma memory, rather than avoiding it, imaginal exposure provides the opportunity for emotional processing.

Third, imaginal exposure helps patients better differentiate between remembering the trauma and being retraumatized by it. Patients with PTSD often report that thinking about the trauma elicits such intense emotions that it makes them feel as if the trauma were happening to them again in that moment. By revisiting the trauma memory in a safe, therapeutic environment, patients learn to discriminate between cognitive representations of threat (i.e., memories of the trauma) and actual threat.

Fourth, imaginal exposure helps patients organize the traumatic memory into a more coherent narrative, which has been associated with symptom improvement (Foa et al., 1995). Fifth, imaginal exposure also promotes differentiation between the traumatic experience and similar stimuli that have become associated with trauma. This differentiation helps patients view the trauma as a specific occurrence, thereby disconfirming the perception that the world is entirely dangerous and the perception that they are unable to cope with stress (being incompetent).

Processing occurs immediately following imaginal exposure and involves discussing the experience of revisiting the trauma memory, with a focus on new learning and changed beliefs or perspectives. Processing is less structured than other components of PE. Therapists first provide positive feedback to reinforce the patient's courage and willingness to approach the trauma memory and to experience distress. Highlighting the patient's ability to remain emotionally engaged during the revisiting helps enhance the patient's sense of self-efficacy. Having monitored the patient's SUDS ratings periodically (approximately every 5 minutes) during the imaginal exposure, therapists may comment on any reduction in distress that was observed either within the imaginal exposure or compared with prior sessions. Attending to patterns observed in the patient's SUDS ratings encourages the patient to consider the meaning of distress reductions and adjust their beliefs about the consequences of approaching the trauma memory. Processing makes the implicit learning explicit. Asking open-ended questions during processing allows patients to express their thoughts and feelings about the trauma and their reaction to it, as well as to the experience of imaginal exposure, and to discuss any insights that seem important or meaningful. This helps patients articulate and integrate new information and insights into their memory. By focusing on aspects of the memory that are central to the erroneous thoughts that are maintaining the patient's PTSD, processing helps patients develop a more realistic perspective on the meaning of the event and their reaction to it. Thus, processing is an integral component of PE because it helps foster the elaboration and consolidation of the new learning that occurs during imaginal exposure.

EFFICACY OF PROLONGED EXPOSURE

The number of randomized controlled trials (RCTs) supporting the efficacy of PE is larger than for any other PTSD treatment. As a result of the number and quality of these trials, PE has been recognized as a first-line treatment for PTSD in all major clinical practice guidelines (American Psychological Association, 2017; International Society for Traumatic Stress Studies, 2018; National Institute for Health and Care Excellence, 2018; VA/DoD, 2017). For the purpose of this review, treatments are considered PE if they include all three of the main components of PE: psychoeducation, in vivo exposure, and imaginal exposure. In PE, imaginal and in vivo exposure are delivered concurrently. Treatment programs wherein imaginal exposure and in vivo exposure are delivered sequentially are also included in this review and are referred to as *modified PE*.

Early Exposure Therapies and Initial Trials of PE

Early studies of exposure therapy for PTSD were focused on variants of imaginal exposure. The first two controlled trials found support for the efficacy of "implosive" (flooding) therapy among veterans compared with waitlist (Keane et al., 1989) and VA treatment as usual (N. Cooper & Clum, 1989). The flooding protocol used in these studies involves the therapist guiding the patient through graduated imaginal exposure to trauma-related scenes. A similar exposure protocol was later found to be more efficacious than counseling-as-usual among veterans with PTSD (Boudewyns & Hyer, 1990).

The first three RCTs of PE were conducted with civilian women with PTSD related to sexual assault. These trials all tested PE in comparison with alternate treatment approaches that were considered more established treatments for PTSD at that time, including *stress inoculation training* (SIT) and *cognitive restructuring* (CR), either alone or in combination. In the very first trial, Foa et al. (1991) found that SIT was superior to supportive counseling (SC) and waitlist, but not PE, in reducing PTSD severity. Analyses of clinically significant PTSD reductions and change in PTSD diagnosis showed that improvements from PE fell in between those of SIT and SC at posttreatment. Intriguingly, by the 3-month follow-up assessment, the effects of PE appeared slightly greater than the effects of SIT. In the second trial, Foa, Dancu, et al. (1999) hypothesized that given the efficacy of PE and SIT as individual treatments, combining PE with SIT would result in superior outcomes relative to either treatment alone. Contrary to hypothesis, the results showed that PE, SIT, and PE + SIT were all superior to waitlist, but that they were not significantly different from each other in reducing PTSD severity. However, the effect size for PE was larger than for the other treatments (Foa, Dancu, et al., 1999). In the third and largest of the three trials, Foa et al. (2005) tested whether adding CR to PE would improve outcomes relative to PE alone. Contrary to hypothesis again, although both PE and PE + CR were superior to waitlist, adding CR to PE did not improve PTSD outcomes relative to PE alone. These first three RCTs established PE as an efficacious treatment for PTSD in women with sexual assault–related PTSD. These studies also showed that combining multiple efficacious treatment approaches may not yield additional benefit.

Efficacy of PE in Civilians

The early trials of PE were led by the developer of PE, Edna Foa, who has continued to study the efficacy of PE in numerous RCTs. However, a notable strength of the large body of research that supports PE is that a majority of the RCTs have been led by independent research groups around the world, thus minimizing the risk of researcher allegiance effects. In addition, PE has been found efficacious in studies of civilians from around the world and in numerous clinical settings. Results from these numerous RCTs support the efficacy of PE in reducing PTSD among civilians with mixed trauma (Fonzo et al., 2017) and women sexual assault survivors compared with waitlist (Cahill et al., 2009; Difede et al., 2007; Foa, Dancu, et al., 1999; Foa et al., 1991; Keane et al., 1989; Resick et al., 2002) and treatment-as-usual (Asukai et al., 2010), with very few exceptions (Foa, Dancu, et al., 1999; McDonagh et al., 2005).

PE has also demonstrated efficacy in RCTs that have compared PE with nonspecific active control conditions. A modified version of PE (imaginal and in vivo exposure implemented sequentially rather than concurrently) with and without CR led to significantly greater PTSD reduction than relaxation training among civilians with mixed trauma (Marks et al., 1998). The same result was found in a later study comparing standard PE with relaxation training in civilians with mixed trauma (Markowitz et al., 2015). Studies of PE have found it to be more efficacious than treatment-as-usual among Japanese civilians with mixed trauma (Asukai et al., 2010) and Australian civilians with mixed trauma (Bryant et al., 2003). Foa et al. (1991) did not find PE to be superior to supportive counseling in reducing PTSD symptoms. This trial was small ($n = 10$–14 per condition), which likely limited power to detect treatment effects. However, the null finding is consistent with that of McDonagh et al. (2005) that found no significant differences between PE and *present-centered therapy* (PCT), an active non-trauma-focused supportive counseling condition among women survivors of childhood sexual abuse.

Several studies have also compared PE with other active PTSD treatments. These types of studies are challenging, in that it can be difficult to attain a large enough sample size to test for differential efficacy with sufficient statistical power. Nonetheless, some studies have found PE to be superior even to other active PTSD treatments. One RCT found that modified PE was superior to both relaxation training and eye-movement desensitization and reprocessing (EMDR) in reducing PTSD severity among civilians with mixed trauma–related PTSD (Taylor et al., 2003). Similarly, PE was found to be efficacious with and without a cognitive enhancer (de Kleine et al., 2012) and superior to waitlist, but not EMDR, in reducing PTSD among Dutch civilians with PTSD related to mixed trauma and comorbid psychosis (van den Berg et al., 2015). Most other civilian trials have found PE to be similarly efficacious as other active PTSD treatments, including SIT (Foa, Dancu, et al., 1999; Foa et al., 1991), cognitive processing therapy (CPT; Resick et al., 2002), and EMDR (Rothbaum et al., 2005) among women rape survivors, and imagery rescripting among Norweigan civilians in an inpatient setting (Langkaas et al., 2017). Similarly, modified PE was found to be as efficacious as cognitive behavioral therapy (CBT) that included exposure among refugees in Sweden (Paunovic & Öst, 2001), and PE combined with SIT was similarly efficacious to EMDR among Australian civilians with mixed trauma (C. Lee et al., 2002). PE was also found to be noninferior to interpersonal psychotherapy, which is an active non-trauma-focused treatment (Markowitz et al., 2015). Overall, this pattern was summarized by a meta-analysis showing that PE was associated with large effect sizes compared with waitlist control conditions, medium effect sizes compared with nonspecific active controls, and small or no differences among active treatments (Powers et al., 2010).

Efficacy of PE in Military Samples

The first trials of PE in a military sample showed that PE led to significantly greater reductions in PTSD severity than PCT among women veterans and active-duty military personnel (Bryant et al., 2003; Schnurr et al., 2007). Subsequent trials have demonstrated the efficacy of PE in men and women veterans. One trial found PE was superior to PCT in military veterans from the wars in Afghanistan and Iraq (S. A. M. Rauch, King, et al., 2015), and another found PE to be superior to treatment-as-usual among Israeli veterans (Nacasch et al., 2015). Exceptions to this pattern included research showing that, although efficacious, PE was not significantly superior to minimal attention, comprising weekly 30-minute phone calls among veterans (Yehuda et al., 2014) or to PCT or relaxation training among older veterans (Thorp et al., 2019). In the first RCT of PE among men and women active-duty military personnel with PTSD, PE delivered in daily sessions over 2 to 3 weeks was more efficacious than minimal attention (weekly 15-minute phone calls), and PE delivered in once-weekly sessions over 8 weeks was noninferior to PCT delivered once-weekly over 8 weeks (Foa et al., 2018). Similar to studies of other first-line PTSD treatments in military samples, the effect sizes for PE in this trial were smaller than is typically seen in civilian trials. Critical reviews of the efficacy of evidence-based psychotherapies (EBPs) in treating PTSD among military samples highlighted the room for improvement in treatment outcomes (Steenkamp et al., 2015).

PE Across Race/Ethnicity and Gender

The intersectionality of race/ethnicity, gender, and class is an important factor in examining the development of PTSD as well as the treatment of PTSD including PE. Additional research is needed to increase methodological rigor and provide insight and understanding of these influences and how they may intersect among populations exposed to additional harms that drive poorer mental health outcomes. In addition, research is needed to determine whether cultural adaptations to EBPs yield superior engagement or clinical outcomes. A strength of PE lies in the individualized protocol and treatment process that is determined by the specific patient presenting for care, allowing for culturally competent clinicians to use PE across a wide range of patient populations (S. A. M. Rauch et al., 2019). In addition, diverse patient populations have been represented in many PE trials conducted to date with African American/ Black patients well represented in some trials but other groups often underrepresented (American Psychological Association, 2017; Benuto et al., 2020). Individual characteristics of the patient, including their experiences of and adaptations to oppression as well as the impact of their ethnic, racial, and gender identity on the trauma before, during, and after the event are always relevant in PE. A solid understanding of ethnic, racial, and gender oppression, both historical and current, is important for PE therapists to work with diverse populations effectively and, for example, to collaborate effectively when identifying safe versus unsafe in vivo exposure or adaptive versus maladaptive hypervigilance in various contexts. Williams et al. (2014) provided an excellent presentation of cultural issues for providers to be aware of, as well as cultural adaptations that may improve engagement or outcomes in PE with diverse patients. As noted in the preface of this book, McClendon et al. (2020) found in a review of PTSD treatment research to date that race/ethnicity did not impact magnitude of change but may impact initiation and retention.

Further, recent advances focusing on the impact of race-based trauma suggest that the impacts of systemic racism can lead to PTSD and related mental health sequalae issues (Bryant-Davis & Ocampo, 2005; Carlson et al., 2018; Carter, 2007). More refined examination is warranted to determine how racism influences the development of PTSD and what interventions may be most effective.

Modifications to PE

Given the large evidence base supporting standard PE, a logical next step is to evaluate whether PE retains its efficacy when modified or integrated with other programs to better meet the needs of a given PTSD population or clinical setting. Although PTSD is commonly comorbid with substance use disorders, clinical lore has long suggested that trauma-focused treatments should be withheld from individuals with comorbid substance use disorders to prevent clinical worsening. However, given the interrelationship between PTSD symptoms and substance use (i.e., substance use is often used as a coping strategy to manage PTSD symptoms), recent trials have tested concurrent and integrated treatment programs that combine PE with approaches that target substance use. Among civilians with PTSD and comorbid alcohol dependence, naltrexone and medication counseling with and without PE were equally effective in reducing PTSD severity (Foa, Gillihan, & Bryant, 2013), although PE showed an advantage on drinking outcomes at the 6-month follow-up (Coffey et al., 2016; Foa, Gillihan, & Bryant, 2013). Coffey et al. (2016) found that PE, with or without motivational enhancement, was superior to a health information control condition in reducing PTSD severity, and that all groups significantly reduced substance use. In both trials, there was no evidence of symptom worsening, indicating that PE is safe and effective when delivered to PTSD patients with substance-use disorder.

A CBT program called Concurrent Treatment of PTSD and Substance Use Disorders Using Prolonged Exposure (COPE; Mills et al., 2012) has been studied in several trials. COPE plus treatment-as-usual was found to be superior to treatment-as-usual alone in reducing PTSD severity, and both groups showed reductions in substance use among civilians with mixed trauma (Mills et al., 2012). Another civilian trial found that COPE and relapse prevention training were both superior to active monitoring in reducing substance use, but that COPE outperformed both groups in reducing PTSD severity (Ruglass et al., 2017). This pattern was recently replicated in a veteran sample; COPE and relapse prevention were not significantly different on the reduction of substance-use severity, but COPE was superior to relapse prevention in reducing PTSD severity (Back et al., 2019). Similarly, not only did veterans who received COPE or Seeking Safety significantly reduce their alcohol use, but those who received COPE experienced significantly greater reductions in PTSD severity (Norman et al., 2019).

One pilot RCT tested a treatment that integrates PE with a treatment for borderline personality disorder (BPD) called *dialectic behavior therapy* (DBT; Linehan et al., 2006). This combined treatment, DBT + PE, was associated with significantly greater reduction in PTSD severity and self-injurious behavior compared with DBT alone among women who had received DBT alone and met BPD-related stability criteria (Harned et al., 2014).

Research has also sought to determine whether PE can be modified for more efficient delivery, without compromising its efficacy. One such program is *PE for primary care*, which involves four 30-minute sessions of PE delivered by behavioral health consultants working in integrated primary care settings. PE for primary care has been found efficacious in reducing PTSD among active-duty military relative to minimal control and shows effectiveness in veterans (Cigrang et al., 2017). PE delivered in 60-minute sessions was found to be as efficacious as it was when delivered in the standard 90-minute sessions (Nacasch et al., 2015). Although this trial was not sufficiently powered for noninferiority ($N = 39$), the efficacy of 60-minute PE sessions was recently tested in a large RCT (Foa, Zandberg, et al., 2019) and the preliminary results indicate noninferiority between the two conditions (Foa et al., 2020). As noted above, PE delivered in daily sessions was found to be noninferior to PE delivered in weekly sessions (Foa et al., 2018). Finally, PE has also been found efficacious when delivered through a self-guided online program with therapist facilitation (McLean et al., 2020).

Efficacy of PE With Comorbidities

PTSD is associated with the highest rate of psychiatric comorbidity of all the psychiatric disorders save for depression. Patients rarely present with PTSD without additional psychiatric problems and associated symptoms. Depression, anxiety, substance use, and symptoms such as dissociation and elevated anger are all common in PTSD samples. Fortunately, PE has been studied in a wide range of PTSD patient populations, and many studies have examined the effects of PE not only on PTSD, but also on symptoms of other disorders and associated problems. As a result, much is known about the breadth and depth of PE's efficacy across patient populations and problem areas.

The most frequently assessed secondary outcome is typically depressive symptoms. PE has been found effective in reducing depressive symptoms in countless trials (Asukai et al., 2010; Foa, Dancu, et al., 1999; Foa & Rothbaum, 1998; Foa et al., 1991, 2005; Foa, Yusko, et al., 2013; Marks et al., 1998; Nacasch et al., 2011; Paunovic & Öst, 2001; Resick et al., 2002; Rothbaum et al., 2005; Taylor et al., 2003). Moreover, PE has also been found effective in reducing PTSD symptoms among patients with comorbid depression (Hagenaars et al., 2010). Patients with current major depression, past major depression, and no history of major depression all benefit equally from PE. One study even found that those with greater depressive symptoms at pretreatment had greater improvement in PTSD symptoms during treatment than those with lower depression (Rizvi et al., 2009). Clearly, the presence of comorbid depression is not a contraindication to PE treatment. However, in cases where major depression is the primary disorder that is causing the greatest distress and dysfunction (e.g., depression significantly interferes with PE engagement), clinicians should consider targeting depressive symptoms first. Similarly, when patients are at imminent high risk for suicide, clinicians should first provide crisis management.

Because of concerns about substance-use exacerbation, treatment studies for PTSD traditionally excluded patients with comorbid substance use disorders. However, as noted above, several studies have now demonstrated that PE is efficacious in reducing PTSD among patients with comorbid alcohol substance use disorders. Patients with comorbid BPD have also traditionally been excluded from PTSD trials. However, pretreatment levels of trait/state dissociation, depersonalization, and numbing (common features of BPD) were not related to PTSD symptom improvement or dropout from PE (Feeny et al., 2002; Harned et al., 2012). These findings contradict the idea that dissociation reduces the efficacy of PE by limiting emotional engagement (e.g., Jaycox & Foa, 1996). One study found that individuals with high dissociation were more likely to meet criteria for PTSD (69%) at follow-up than those with low dissociation (10%; Hagenaars et al., 2010). When treating patients who dissociate under distress, clinicians should discuss a plan for modifying exposure or providing grounding techniques as described in the PE protocol. Although some research supports the use of emotional regulation skills prior to imaginal exposure (Cloitre et al., 2012), the utility of adding this additional procedure to standard PE is unknown. As noted earlier, studies integrating PE with DBT have found that this approach is effective in reducing PTSD among women with comorbid BPD and recent or imminent serious intentional self-injury (Harned et al., 2012), or both. Traumatic brain injury (TBI) is also frequently comorbid with PTSD and is common among active military personnel and veterans. However, studies have shown that those with mild to moderate TBI still benefit from PE (Ragsdale & Voss Horrell, 2016; Sripada et al., 2013; G. K. Wolf et al., 2015).

PE has been shown to improve general anxiety (Foa, Dancu, et al., 1999; Foa et al., 2005; Marks et al., 1998; Nacasch et al., 2011; Power et al., 2002; Rothbaum et al., 2005; Schnurr et al., 2007), trauma-related guilt (Resick et al., 2002), and anger (Cahill et al., 2003). PE has been associated with decreased physical health difficulties compared with waitlist, and these improvements persisted at 12 months posttreatment (S. A. M. Rauch et al., 2009). PE has a broad and significant impact on the lives of those with PTSD by reducing both PTSD severity and associated symptoms as well as improving overall functioning (Foa, Dancu, et al., 1999; Foa et al., 2005; Foa, Yusko, et al., 2013; Power et al., 2002; Shemesh et al., 2011).

Limitations of PE

As noted above, PE has shown efficacy across a wide range of PTSD presentations and comorbidities and is supported as a first-line treatment (American Psychiatric Association, 2017). As with all PTSD treatments available, there are limitations to PE related to access, retention, and remission. A comprehensive review of these issues is beyond the scope of this book, although a brief mention is provided. With regard to access, most people suffering with PTSD do not have access to providers who are trained in PE. Socioeconomic and geographic factors contribute but lack of provider training is also a significant issue. In addition, even among trained providers, PE is underutilized, as training does not address the logistic and organizational barriers to using PE (e.g., lack of weekly 90-minute appointments) that can limit adoption and sustained use (Borah et al., 2013; Hepner et al., 2018; Wilk et al., 2013). As a result, PE is often provided only in specialty mental health settings, thus creating barriers to care because most patients receive mental health care in primary care or community-based settings. PE for primary care (PE-PC) has been developed to address this access issue and has demonstrated efficacy (S. A. M. Rauch et al., 2017; see also Chapter 13, this volume). Finally, as discussed in Chapter 12, in clinical practice up to half of patients do not complete PE and some of those who complete may not meet full remission (Kehle-Forbes et al., 2016), highlighting the importance of continued research on augmentation strategies to make PE more efficient, reduce dropout, and improve outcomes.

PART **II** NEUROSCIENCE METHODS FOR CLINICIANS

3 NEUROSTEROIDS, CORTISOL, AND OTHER NEUROCHEMICALS

Recent advances have shown that many neurochemicals are involved in both the development and maintenance of posttraumatic stress disorder (PTSD) symptoms as well as its effective treatment. These neurochemical actors can enhance or inhibit brain processes to convey increased or decreased risk following trauma as well as increased or decreased response to treatment. Timing, location, and dose of neurochemicals further complicate examination, such that the same chemical when provided at a different time (acute trauma phase vs. chronic PTSD), at a different site in the brain, or at a different dose can have opposing effects. In addition, most of the research to date focuses only on the direct actions of specific chemicals and systems, even though all neurochemicals are present in the brain concurrently, interacting across systems. Finally, no single neurochemical process has been uniformly supported to produce PTSD or be related to PTSD across all people with PTSD. As noted by Rasmusson and Pineles (2018), this means that multiple systems and neurochemical processes are involved with variations in those processes between individuals, contributing to the heterogeneity we see in how PTSD presents, sometimes referred to in neuroscience as *phenotypes*.

In their review of neurobiological factors in PTSD, Rasmusson and Pineles (2018) concluded that individual variation in brain systems at the molecular

https://doi.org/10.1037/0000242-003
Retraining the Brain: Applied Neuroscience in Exposure Therapy for PTSD,
by S. A. M. Rauch and C. P. McLean

level interact to produce variable phenotypes of PTSD, with some abnormalities offset or amplified by other abnormalities within the system or within related systems involved in stress response. For instance, the hypothalamic–pituitary–adrenal (HPA) axis provides input to the catecholamine system (Eiden, 2013), and these systems may be complementary or opposing in their effects.

This chapter focuses on those systems and chemicals that have the most research findings relevant to PTSD. We aim to relate the amazing developments in our understanding of these neurochemical actors as they apply to prolonged exposure (PE) and its practice in the treatment of PTSD, beginning with a description of the methods of scientific discovery and factors to consider when interpreting neuroscience to provide background for the nonneuroscientist. We then move on to describe how the relevant systems and neurochemicals work in general and discuss recent discoveries of how they may impact PTSD and its treatment using PE, as well as how we can capitalize on these discoveries in order to optimize patient outcomes.

METHODS OF SCIENTIFIC DISCOVERY

When considering the methods of examination of neurochemicals, it is important to know that neurochemical systems are interconnected and responsive to much more than trauma. Indeed, these systems respond to time of day, novelty, social threat, hunger, and the actions of other systems. Methods of collection and examination of stress responsive systems must account for many factors. For instance, sleep and time of day robustly impact the HPA axis, and this will be reflected differently based on whether the method collects saliva, blood, urine, hair, and so forth. In addition, timing of collection following exposure to stress, smoking, food, and so on is also important to know because this will affect response. When collections occur across time of day, diurnal (daily) variations of neurochemicals may overwhelm any variability due to PTSD or treatment status.

For instance, diurnal variation in cortisol, a primary neurochemical involved in stress response, shows generally lower levels in the afternoon and evening. Therefore, studies that stress people in the afternoon may be better able to show system activation compared with studies in the morning. Of note, if a specific stress system is already activated, any additional response may be less apparent, and methods need to account for this variation. For instance, recent research using hair cortisol has shown interesting and promising results as a marker of longer term trauma and stress exposure load but is difficult to interpret within the existing literature. Hair cortisol is a reflection of average stress system responses over a longer time window (months or years) than blood or salivary collections (minutes to hours; Wright et al., 2015).

Previous research has typically used several different methods: (a) diurnal collections of blood, saliva, or urine over a specified time period (e.g., saliva collected every 2 hours over 2 days); (b) collections at specific times of day (i.e., cortisol awakening collections); (c) salivary or blood collections in response to specified challenge tasks; and (d) cerebrospinal fluid (CSF) collections through lumbar puncture at specified times of day. All these methods have strengths and weaknesses that should be acknowledged in interpretation. Diurnal collections are cumbersome for participants, leading to noncompliance with procedures and potential uncertainty of data quality without specific verifications. For instance, ideal saliva collection involves (a) making sure timing is precisely directed (e.g., get the first saliva prior to sitting up); (b) that saliva is not contaminated by eating, drinking, or smoking during the collection period; (c) that it is stored in accordance with standards across patients (e.g., either everyone refrigerates or does not); and (d) that there is enough of the saliva to run the tests (e.g., if the patient is dehydrated there may not be enough saliva to collect). However, precision of collections may vary (e.g., the patient may brush their teeth prior to salivary cortisol collection) and storage methods may vary (e.g., in how long before the collection was refrigerated). In addition, it is difficult to covary out the many daily life stressors and factors that influence neuroactive chemicals that introduce "noise." For instance, exams or changes in sleep patterns for students or shift workers involved in research can greatly alter the system responses. For cortisol awakening response (change in cortisol concentration that occurs in the first hour after waking from sleep), previous methodological variability made it difficult to know whether the measure was consistently collected across studies and laboratories. Recent consensus guidelines are working to address this issue (Stalder et al., 2016) through standardized methods of collection and verifications of collection.

For challenge tasks, such as the Trier Social Stress Test (Birkett, 2011) or script-driven imagery (Orr et al., 2012), it is often unclear whether the task and collections are standardized across studies. Variability related to the specific challenge task (aversiveness of stressor across laboratories, etc.) occurs. In addition, what is considered a stress task may not be a stress to the specific neurochemical system that is targeted for examination. As an example, if perceived control is high when confronted with a stressful situation, HPA axis (see the next section for system description) activation, as measured in cortisol release, is less robust than when control is not perceived (Bollini et al., 2004). In addition, variance is introduced by the specific time of day for administration. Finally, stress response systems require time to activate and the amount of time required varies based on system and response. Further, the full response cycle may also require time leading to long study sessions. For HPA axis response to stressors, activation often requires at least 30 to 45 minutes for peak activation and another 30 to 45 minutes to capture return to baseline, even for a brief activation task (e.g., a 1-minute trauma script). With all the system inputs and influencers, methods are very important to ensure that what the researchers are seeing reflects what they believe it reflects. As a final point, even when all of the system inputs and influencers are known, established studies show that the internal context (previous genetic, biological, and learning history) and external context (smoking, medications, and eating prior to examination) heavily influence system responses (Rasmusson & Pineles, 2018). Thus, precision in methodology is critical.

HYPOTHALAMIC-PITUITARY-ADRENAL (HPA) AXIS

The HPA axis is one of the primary systems that has been implicated in the development, maintenance, and treatment of PTSD. As a key system involved in stress response, many believe this system might orchestrate the body's responses that lead to PTSD following trauma, with cortisol providing signals to the brain and body activating the stress and trauma response.

How the HPA Axis Works

The HPA axis involves several neuroactive chemicals and structures that work in feedback loops to activate and deactivate response. As a loop, we begin with the hypothalamus receiving an input (e.g., an environmental stressor) that requires system response. Upon exposure to an activating stimulus, the hypothalamus releases corticotrophin-releasing hormone (CRH) and vasopressin that act on the anterior pituitary as a signal to release adrenocorticotropic hormone (ACTH) that then acts on the adrenal glands (on top of the kidneys) to synthesize and release cortisol. The cortisol that is released then acts as a brake on the release of CRH from the hypothalamus and ACTH from the pituitary in a negative feedback loop to turn off the system response (see Figure 3.1).

In a recent review, Rasmusson and Pineles (2018) summarized several of the key feedback loops of the HPA axis that regulate activation and inhibition in the system and are relevant to PTSD. The most explored feedback loop involves cortisol activation of glucocorticoid receptors (GRs) in the hypothalamus and pituitary gland to inhibit release of CRH and ACTH. This leads to slowing down of the release of cortisol by the adrenal gland and turning off the system

FIGURE 3.1. Hypothalamic-Pituitary-Adrenal Axis System

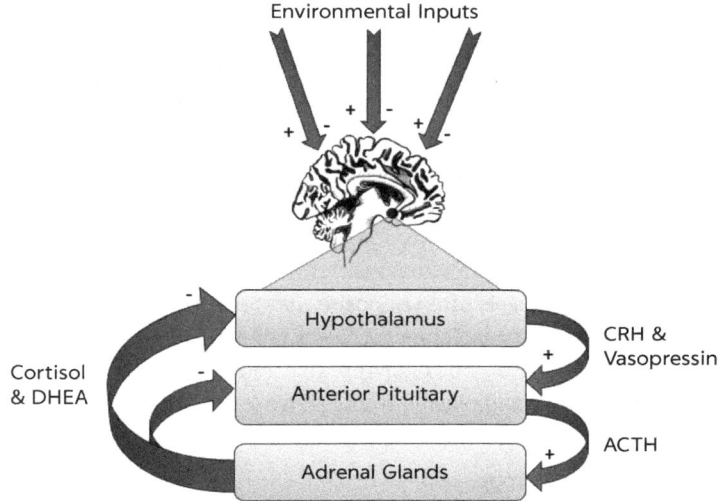

Note. ACTH = adrenocorticotropic hormone; CRH = corticotrophin-releasing hormone; DHEA = dehydroepiandrosterone.

activation. A second loop is driven by the release of dehydroepiandrosterone (DHEA) from the adrenal gland as it releases cortisol. DHEA speeds the metabolism of cortisol to its metabolites. A third loop involves *FK506*-binding protein 51 (*FKBP5*) that regulates GR sensitivity within peripheral and central nervous system cells where GR activation reduces GR sensitivity (Binder, 2009). The last characterized feedback loop occurs a bit later and involves allopregnanolone (see the later section on sex hormones) that peaks about an hour after stressor exposure. Allopregnanolone facilitates inhibition of CRH and ACTH release. Abnormalities across these loops have differing impacts (Rasmusson & Pineles, 2018). As applied to PTSD, if a given trauma survivor has more allopregnanolone available in the brain in the immediate aftermath of trauma, this is likely to have an anti-anxiety and anti-inflammatory impact that would result in a lower likelihood of PTSD development. High allopregnanolone may occur based not only on individual differences in biological system response but also will differ within a person based on menstrual cycle in women and potentially other factors in men.

Interactions between brain regions involved in cognitive, behavioral, and emotional processing and regulation influence the HPA axis (i.e., King et al., 2009). Experience regulated GR sensitivities in the pituitary gland then produce ACTH in response to CRH. Sex differences in HPA axis function are apparent (Stroud et al., 2002), and psychosocial factors robustly activate the system, including novelty, perceived lack of control or access to coping when confronted with threat, and lack of social support (Dickerson & Kemeny, 2004). Recent reviews provide additional details about the state of the science in HPA axis function (Rasmusson & Pineles, 2018; S. A. M. Rauch, Abelson, et al., 2015).

The HPA axis was one of the first neurobiological abnormalities identified in PTSD and has been subjected to significant study for the past 30 years (Mason et al., 1986, 2002). Equivocal results suggesting both hyper- and hypocortisolemia across studies based on the complexities of the HPA axis and its relationships to other regulatory systems are common. In addition, the high rates of depression in PTSD contribute to inconsistent results, as the impact of depression on HPA axis response is often opposite that found in PTSD. Initial results suggested general hypocortisolemia (or lower general system response) based on diurnal urinary cortisol, but later research found the opposite, and challenge tasks and salivary and plasma studies have led to varied results as well.

What Does This Mean for PTSD and PE?

PTSD is associated with enhanced glucocorticoid negative feedback inhibition (Yehuda et al., 2004) and an attenuated cortisol awakening response (Neylan et al., 2005). In addition, reduced cortisol reactivity to acute stress prior to trauma exposure predicts increased risk for PTSD following trauma exposure (Galatzer-Levy, Steenkamp, et al., 2014), and rape survivors with lower cortisol response in the emergency room had higher risk for developing PTSD than those with higher acute cortisol response (Walsh et al., 2013). Additional neurochemicals have also been examined, such as DHEA, CRH, and so forth, with mixed results (Van Voorhees et al., 2014).

Few studies have examined change in HPA axis function during treatment, and, among studies that have, variations in methods have resulted in significant heterogeneity in results. When examining a single sample of salivary cortisol collected at baseline, and post Session 3 and Session 9, treatment response was associated with reductions in cortisol across treatment (Gerardi et al., 2010). While overall HPA axis activation may be reduced with effective treatment, this does not necessarily relate to the system response during therapy sessions. Specifically, in a study examining cortisol response within each of PE Sessions 3, 6, and 10, veterans who showed less PTSD reduction in treatment (low responders) showed an increase in cortisol during each session across treatment. Thus, patients who responded to treatment did not show an increase in cortisol during their sessions while those who had a lower response to treatment showed increased cortisol across their sessions. Finally, baseline higher cortisol response to a brief (1 to 2 minute) experimental presentation of the target trauma predicted more PTSD reduction with PE (S. A. M. Rauch, King, et al., 2015), but when the baseline presentation of the target trauma stimulus was longer (as would be the case in imaginal exposure), higher cortisol was related to lower response to PE (Norrholm et al., 2016). Together, these results point to PE reducing the system's general response to stressors (e.g., the brief experimental session activation where more cortisol in response to brief scripts is related to better treatment response) but not necessarily altering response to longer exposures to the target trauma as occurs in imaginal exposure in session. When moving to examine general system function using cortisol awakening response (CAR), one study showed increased CAR in high treatment responders (more than 50% reduction in PTSD) compared with low responders, as well as increased CAR in those who received PE as opposed to present centered therapy (S. A. M. Rauch, King, et al., 2015); another study found the opposite result among women (nonresponse was related to higher CAR) and no effect in men (Pacella et al., 2014). These apparently contradictory findings support the importance of considering the impact of sex on cortisol. The pattern of results is likely impacted by low sample size of one sex, meaning the results are driven by just the well-represented sex (Pacella, female $n = 21$; Rauch, male $n = 33$).

Neuropeptide Y (NPY) is a neurotransmitter that is related to coping and resilience that acts on the HPA axis and other stress systems (see the next section on catecholamines). In a study examining PE and minimal attention control, higher plasma NPY, lower DHEA/cortisol (CORT) ratio, lower 24-hour urinary cortisol, and higher bedtime salivary cortisol at pretreatment predicted response to both conditions (Yehuda et al., 2014). This lack of condition effect may be due to low power given small sample size ($N = 52$). Indeed, the large difference in average symptoms reduction across conditions (PE showed 23-point reduction and minimal attention control showed 14-point reduction) suggests that power may have been an issue (Yehuda et al., 2014). Replication with appropriate power to detect a difference is warranted.

On the basis of research showing that hydrocortisone improves extinction learning (Merz et al., 2018), several studies have examined whether cortisol administration or related augmentations are effective at improving response to PE as an exposure-based treatment. In one study, augmentation was associated with greater reduction in total PTSD symptoms compared with placebo (Yehuda et al., 2015), although the authors indicated that this was driven by better retention in the hydrocortisone condition compared with placebo. On examination of possible mechanisms involved in the augmentation effect, Yehuda et al. (2015) examined whether responder status by condition was related to pretreatment glucocorticoid sensitivity and found that responders to hydrocortisone augmentation had the highest glucocorticoid sensitivity of all groups and that this diminished over the course of treatment. Other augmentation trials have targeted increased cortisol availability during PE sessions through administration of dexamethasone and found no augmentation effect and much higher rates of drop from treatment (Maples-Keller, Jovanovic, et al., 2019).

In summary, additional research is needed to clarify the many roles of cortisol, DHEA, DHEAS, and the other HPA axis neurochemicals to clearly delineate how to harness this system for therapeutic benefit. However, changes in the system with effective treatment, including response to personal trauma scripts and CAR have been found—although not consistently.

CATECHOLAMINES

Catecholamines are synthesized in the sympathetic nervous system and adrenal medulla from the amino acid tyrosine. These neurotransmitters modulate the fight or flight reaction in response to acute stressors and include epinephrine (adrenaline), norepinephrine (noradrenaline), dopamine, NPY, and others.

How Catecholamines Work

In response to acute threat/stress, the adrenal medulla synthesizes and releases epinephrine that signals the release of norepinephrine from the locus coeruleus, a nucleus in the pons of the brain stem. These neurotransmitters support the response needed for acute threat and coping and facilitate the processes involved in long-term responses connected to robust emotional memory encoding (Ouyang et al., 2012) and consolidation of fear and trauma memory (Eiden, 2013; Hauer et al., 2014; Matthews et al., 2012; McLaughlin et al., 2015). NPY is a neurotransmitter that is related to coping and resilience that acts on the HPA axis and other stress systems. In this process, NPY then acts as a brake on the release of noradrenaline and other neurotransmitters to bring the system back to baseline (Rasmusson & Pineles, 2018). As a case of system interplay, NPY synthesis is up-regulated by glucocorticoids and testosterone and down-regulated by estradiol, making the interactions between HPA axis and sex hormone function highly relevant to expression of PTSD (Misaki et al., 1992; Zukowska-Grojec, 1995).

In addition to the HPA axis results reported above, Yehuda et al. (2014) found that higher plasma NPY at pretreatment predicted treatment response in both PE and minimal attention control. This lack of condition effect may be due to low power given small sample size ($N = 52$) but still does support that higher NPY at baseline generally supports therapeutic change. As previously suggested, replication with appropriate power to detect conditional differences is warranted.

What Does This Mean for PTSD and PE?

A recent meta-analysis concluded that people with PTSD showed higher nor-epinephrine levels than controls without PTSD but no differences in epineph-rine or dopamine comparing PTSD to controls (Pan et al., 2018). However, the studies reviewed showed significant heterogeneity in methodology and results, suggesting that there may be more specific effects for certain sub-groups that are not apparent when combined across studies. Similarly, in their review, Rasmusson and Pineles (2018) concluded that PTSD is associated with increased norepinephrine levels in brain and blood compared with com-bat exposure alone but that this characterizes only a subpopulation of those with PTSD (Rasmusson & Pineles, 2018). In addition, when reviewing the research relevant to the association of NPY and PTSD diagnostic status, they concluded that men with PTSD showed lower NPY in their blood and cere-brospinal fluid than men with combat exposure and no PTSD (Rasmusson & Pineles, 2018). Gender and trauma type subgroup analyses suggested these relationships may differ by sex and early life versus late trauma exposures (Pan et al., 2018).

In terms of treatment effects, Yehuda et al. (2014) found that baseline NPY predicted therapeutic response to PTSD therapy, suggesting that catechol-amine system responsiveness may impact treatment response. Several studies have looked at the therapeutic effects of medications that act on the catechol-amine system. For instance, prazosin blocks the effects of alpha-1 adrenergic receptors and has shown mixed results in efficacy as a primary treatment for PTSD, with the largest clinical trial to date showing no separation from pla-cebo (Raskind et al., 2018). Some have suggested that prazosin may be ideal for augmentation of PE because it may speed reduction of nightmares and improve sleep (Strawn & Geracioti, 2008). However, in a records review of vet-erans receiving both PE and prazosin or no prazosin, those with the combined prazosin plus PE had significantly less reduction in PTSD over time than those who received PE alone (Myers et al., 2019). Thus, in practice, prazosin does not appear to be adding to the effect of PE.

On the basis of its role as a centrally acting alpha-2 agonist, clonidine has been proposed, and some initial open trials have supported its use for hyper-arousal and vigilance and sleep in PTSD (Strawn & Geracioti, 2008). Additional clinical trials and augmentation studies may be warranted, especially because these symptoms are among those most likely to remain in partial responders to PE.

Although initial studies supported efficacy of propranolol (a centrally acting beta-blocker) for PTSD prevention when administered within hours of trauma exposure, use for PTSD treatment has not been supported (Strawn & Geracioti, 2008). Propranolol was believed to reduce recall of emotional memories, but preclinical studies have not translated to clear clinical treatment outcomes, though research is ongoing.

Tuerk et al. (2018) examined whether combining yohimbine, an alpha-2 andrenergic antagonist, with PE lead to facilitated treatment response. Yohimbine led to higher objective and subjective arousal during the exposure session and to lower trauma-cued heart rate reactivity 1 week later for those who received yohimbine as compared with placebo. The single dose of yohimbine also led to greater between-session habituation and more rapid improvement on depression, but not PTSD, over the course of care visit for those who received yohimbine as compared with placebo (Tuerk et al., 2018).

SEX HORMONES

Sex differences in rates of PTSD posttrauma have led many to examine what factors may contribute to these differences. Allopregnanolone and pregnanolone are neurosteroid sex hormones with multiple key functions. Although they are most well known for their roles within reproduction, they also have key roles in brain neuroprotection and neurogenesis. They have most often been studied in women but are also present and key actors for brain function and mood in men (Reddy, 2010). Together, these neurosteroids produce anxiolytic, analgesic, and anti-aggressive effects through modulation of gamma aminobutyric acid (GABA) receptors (Pineles et al., 2018). As such, they are highly relevant to the development and treatment of PTSD.

Similarly, testosterone is best known for its key role in reproduction and is viewed as a key male sex hormone, although it is present and important for both female and male function (Celec et al., 2015). Testosterone is primarily produced in the testes of men and ovaries of women but is also synthesized in the adrenal gland and even the brain (Dohle et al., 2003; Mellon et al., 2001, 2007). In their review of the impact of testosterone on brain behavioral function, Celec et al. (2015) concluded that, across many studies to date, testosterone shows an anxiolytic effect in both men and women. In addition, administration has demonstrated increased verbal and spatial memory ability for both men and women, although the mechanism of action remains unclear (Celec et al., 2015).

How Hormones Work in the Brain

The actions of sex hormones in the brain have received significant attention, with preclinical research supporting the roles of estradiol and progesterone in fear acquisition, extinction, and retention processes that are highly relevant to the development and treatment of PTSD (Garcia et al., 2018). A recent comprehensive review (Garcia et al., 2018) concluded that among females, higher estradiol was consistently associated with enhanced fear extinction recall and inconsistently associated with better extinction learning and fear acquisition. However, the consistency of results breaks down when research moves from fear learning to clinical translational studies including treatment. This may be due to the complexity of factors involved in treatment, including extended time over which treatment is administered, resulting in normal cyclical hormone patterns, and the like. These factors are many, including whether to dose before or after sessions, whether to dose based on session outcome, what specific hormone or balance of hormones may provide maximum benefit in extinction recall over time, and so forth. Finally, replication of the impact of these hormones in men is also needed. Therefore, additional work is needed to know when and how to dose these potential augmentations to enhance extinction recall in PE.

What Does This Mean for PTSD and PE?

On the basis of their normal functions, sex hormones have long been considered important in the development of PTSD and, more recently, have been raised as potentially relevant to treatment response. In their review of research that has examined the impact of these hormones on fear extinction, Ramusson and Pineles (2018) concluded that higher estradiol is associated with better fear extinction and retention in healthy women and that low estradiol in women with PTSD is associated with poor fear extinction. Allopregnanolone and pregnanolone—often referred together as ALLO—have been negatively and strongly correlated with PTSD severity (Rasmusson & Pineles, 2018). In women and men with PTSD, ALLO concentrations in cerebrospinal fluid are reduced (Rasmusson et al., 2006, 2019) due to a block in ALLO synthesis (Pineles et al., 2018; Rasmusson et al., 2019). Recent research has also shown that higher allopregnanolone at baseline is related to greater PTSD reduction in PE (S. A. M. Rauch et al., 2020a, 2020b).

OXYTOCIN

Oxytocin is a hormone produced in the hypothalamus and sent to the pituitary, where it is expressed into the blood and is involved in bonding and social connection as well as sexual reproduction and childbirth.

How Oxytocin Works in the Brain

Oxytocin has been suggested as a therapeutic agent to promote prosocial behavior, connection, positive social memory, and so forth. In addition, release of oxytocin modulates the HPA axis response to stress and assists in return to baseline following stress (Donadon et al., 2018).

What Does This Mean for PTSD and PE?

In a review of literature to date, Donandon et al. (2018) concluded that both trauma exposure and PTSD were related to lower endogenous oxytocin and that administration studies produced mixed results, possibly due to methodological variations and to not specifying those patients with deficits that oxytocin may most robustly affect. Additional more specified (directed at those with deficits and collected during therapy when its impact may be most relevant) examination of the role of oxytocin during therapy is needed as the robust findings of social support facilitating natural recovery and treatment response suggest this mechanism (Price et al., 2013). Because of the role of oxytocin interacting with the HPA axis, administration of oxytocin produces anxiolytic effects and has been suggested as a therapeutic agent to compensate for negative feedback inhibition when present in PTSD (for a review, see Donadon et al., 2018).

BRAIN-DERIVED NEUROTROPHIC FACTOR

Brain-derived neurotrophic factor (BDNF) is a protein expressed within and outside the limbic system that plays a critical role in neuronal survival and plasticity in the hippocampus and is especially relevant to learning and memory (Andero & Ressler, 2012). BDNF is involved in fear and stress responses and critical periods of brain development (for a review, see J. K. Miller et al., 2017).

How BDNF Works in the Brain

Of relevance to the development and treatment of PTSD, BDNF facilitates learning by supporting the growth and maturation of nerve cells—thus helping to encode any new learning. Efforts to increase the levels of BDNF expression in the brain to help facilitate psychotherapies, such as PE, have found that several medications as well as exercise are effective (Liu & Nusslock, 2018). Additional discussion of BDNF can be found in Chapter 7.

What Does This Mean for PTSD and PE?

Animal studies support that higher availability of BDNF in the hippocampus facilitates fear extinction (Andero & Ressler, 2012; J. K. Miller et al., 2017). Given the key role that extinction learning plays in PE, investigators began to examine ways to increase availability of BDNF prior to or during exposure therapy. Powers et al. (2015) found that adding exercise prior to PE sessions enhanced reductions in PTSD symptoms compared with patients who received PE alone. In addition, those patients who received exercise had significantly higher BDNF than those who received PE alone (Powers et al., 2015).

CONCLUSION

Many neurochemical actors are relevant to the development and treatment of PTSD. Recent research advances in translational neuroscience have contributed to new considerations of how PE, and other treatments, work in the brain and how we might facilitate treatments to work more efficiently and effectively (Olff & van Zuiden, 2017). Continued work is needed to further clarify the roles that these neurochemicals and systems play in PTSD, but providers of PE can use the current chapter in concert with the following chapters, which provide additional specification of the most promising applications of neuroscience to PE practice, to begin to gain insight into the systems involved.

4

IMAGING

For the past 30 years, many have been heralding neuroimaging methodology as the most promising approach for new discovery across neuroscience. Neuroimaging research has indeed provided new insights into the processes involved in posttraumatic stress disorder (PTSD) development and effective treatment approaches, including prolonged exposure (PE). Although this powerful tool has provided numerous new insights, the promise of being able to provide a "picture" of PTSD has not yet been realized (Im et al., 2017), and many researchers now have pulled back from this idea, noting heterogeneity of PTSD (Galatzer-Levy & Bryant, 2013) and difficulties in standardization of imaging methodology across scanners and procedures as well as cost. In addition, PTSD is a heterogeneous disorder that will likely have multiple presentations. As a tool, the clinical field is still quite far from being able to use imaging to provide case differentials at the level of the individual patient, although some potential use cases are described. In this chapter, we review and summarize current methodologies within neuroimaging in the areas where they may inform PTSD development and treatment. We then review these advances and explain what they mean for the status of the field today, as well as next steps. Finally, we discuss how the tools of neuroimaging might inform clinical care.

https://doi.org/10.1037/0000242-004
Retraining the Brain: Applied Neuroscience in Exposure Therapy for PTSD,
by S. A. M. Rauch and C. P. McLean

METHODS FOR SCIENTIFIC DISCOVERY

A complete review of all possible neuroimaging methods is beyond the scope of this chapter. A recent special issue that was focused on traumatic brain injury and application to PTSD provided an excellent general review of imaging methodologies (Prasad et al., 2012). We focus our review on recent methods that have been used effectively to provide insight into the brain structure and function involved in the development and treatment of PTSD. Imaging methods can be broken into three large categories: structural imaging, functional imaging, and metabolic imaging.

Structural Imaging

Structural imaging can be used to examine the anatomy and differential diffusion (e.g., size, white matter density) of brain structures across different patients and healthy populations. Magnetic resonance imaging (MRI) and computed tomography (CAT) scans are the most common specifically structural scans. These scanners and analytic techniques can be used to find frank structural difference in size of specific brain structures within a population, such as the work described below examining hippocampal volume and looking for specific lesions or injuries. Most recently, these techniques have been used to examine white matter integrity, connectivity, and thickness.

Functional Imaging

Functional imaging examines activations and deactivations in the brain over time. The most common functional imaging technique used in research to explore PTSD is functional magnetic resonance imaging (fMRI). fMRI relies on blood-oxygen-level-dependent imaging, usually referred to as BOLD imaging. This technique models activations in the brain that are based on the patient being placed in a powerful magnet. The system then models the magnetic responses from hemoglobin in the blood, showing where concentrations of blood are higher or lower in the brain, and infers that those areas receiving more blood are more activated, because blood is needed to provide glucose— the fuel for the brain. Because functional imaging measures change over time, it is critical to know what the patient is doing to interpret any scan results. Typically, studies using these techniques have focused on task-related activations. Such tasks can vary widely in the intent to activate certain regions. For instance, fear learning tasks will often present threat stimuli (e.g., an image of an angry face) on a screen inside the scanner in order to see how the brain responds to threat. Alternatively, a mindfulness or breathing task would be expected to show very different activations. In addition, there are between-laboratory variabilities within each task. More recently, resting state scans, where the person being scanned is asked to focus on a cross for the duration of the scan, have become a prominent tool based on the ability to more consistently compare across laboratories and patient types. Although this has led to interesting findings and advances, these techniques are always challenged by the complexity of the human brain and the fact that patients vary in what they "do" when asked to rest. For instance, a PTSD patient when asked to stare at a cross may experience flashbacks that would alter brain activation patterns.

Modeling and analytic methods used in fMRI have improved greatly over the years of use. We are now better able to show more precise changes in time and even better images of deeper brain processes and connections between structures of the brain. More recent techniques that better account for the dynamic nature of brain function, such as connectivity analysis and network analysis, are providing additional new insights.

Metabolic Imaging

Metabolic imaging methods provide another view of brain function over time through the lens of specific uptake, metabolism, or concentrations of neurotransmitters or other neurochemicals. The three metabolic imaging techniques most often used are positron emission tomography (PET), single-photon emission computerized tomography (SPECT), and magnetic resonance spectroscopy (MRS). Brain consumption of glucose and oxygen (the brain's fuel) are the most commonly examined metabolic imaging targets. In addition, these techniques can use radioactive tracers to examine other specific neurochemicals and receptor densities, such as those related to inflammation, dementia, or other brain function or dysfunction (Prasad et al., 2019). The goal with all brain imaging is to provide a window into brain structure or function in vivo that previously was only possible to examine postmortem. New methods of combining across different imagining techniques, such as multimodal neuroimaging, and the use of machine learning to combine large imaging datasets to maximize the ability to discriminate recovery from PTSD following trauma exposure are now being explored (Galatzer-Levy, Karstoft, et al., 2014; Im et al., 2017).

What Does This Mean for PTSD?

Consistent findings have begun to take shape across neuroimaging studies that illuminate differences between those with PTSD compared with non-PTSD healthy control brain structure and function, as well as compared with other disorders. Figure 4.1 shows an updated model of the neurocircuitry of PTSD, presented by S. A. M. Rauch, Abelson, et al. (2015) in their review of neuroimaging of PTSD and building on previous neurocircuitry models (S. L. Rauch et al., 1998), as it relates to three key processes: emotion generation and response, emotion regulation and modulation, and contextualization. *Emotion generation and response* includes activating the emotion regions of the brain, as well as recognition of environmental emotional stimuli and initial interpretation. *Emotion regulation and modulation* includes sustaining emotional activation over time and increasing or decreasing an emotional activation. Finally, *contextualization* includes placing an emotional activation within a specific place and time or leaving it as a general activation across different times and places. These three processes are critical in the development, maintenance, and treatment of PTSD as described below. Emotion generation and response involves the dorsal anterior cingulate (dACC), insula, and amygdala. Emotion regulation and modulation includes the ventromedial prefrontal cortex (vmPFC), rostral anterior cingulate cortex (rACC), and hippocampus (Rougemont-Bücking et al., 2011). Contextualization critically uses the hippocampus, interacting with both emotion generation and regulation processes. Additional brain regions and processes are involved, but the heuristic model below provides a useful guide for the processes most relevant to the development and treatment of PTSD.

In human models of PTSD, the amygdala is central to threat detection, fear expression, and fear learning, and the dACC facilitates expression of conditioned fear along with the amygdala (Milad et al., 2007, 2009). The insula is involved in the acquisition of fear learning, threat anticipation, and

FIGURE 4.1. Neurocircuitry Model of PTSD (S. A. M. Rauch, Abelson, et al., 2015)

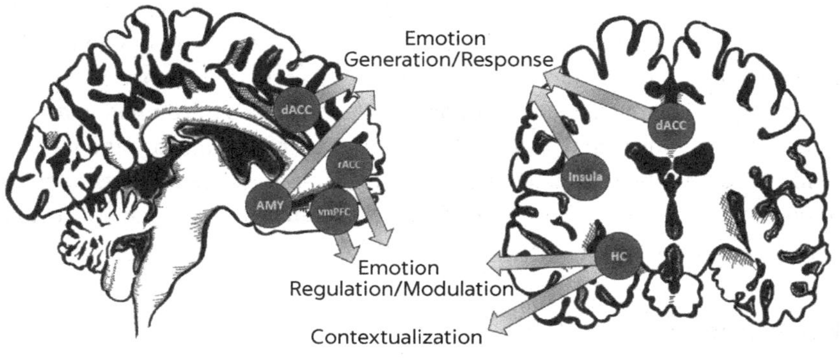

Note. AMY = amygdala; dACC = dorsal anterior cingulate; HC = hippocampus; rACC = rostral anterior cingulate cortex; vmPFC = ventromedial prefrontal cortex.

introspective somatic sensation of emotions (Linnman et al., 2011). As illustrated in Figure 4.1, the amygdala and the dACC process incoming stimuli and provide that information to the hypothalamus, basal ganglia, and brain stem to initiate threat responses and simultaneously activate the hypothalamic–pituitary–adrenal (HPA) axis (see Chapter 3). Whereas structural studies have produced conflicting results showing both increased and decreased volumes of amygdala related to PTSD (Woon & Hedges, 2009), a review of PET and fMRI studies concluded that PTSD patients showed increased activation in dACC and amygdala as compared with control adults (Hayes et al., 2012). With regard to the insula, Hughes and Shin (2011) concluded that increased insula activation is related to PTSD as compared with trauma exposed controls, although this may not be specific to PTSD because this increased activation has also been found in other anxiety disorders (Etkin & Wager, 2007).

PTSD patients also show hypoactivation in the vmPFC, and the level of hypoactivation is related to the level of hyperactivation in the amygdala (Hayes et al., 2012). In a recent review of neuroimaging, Negreira and Abdallah (2019) concluded that trauma priming paradigm studies demonstrated hypoactivation of vmPFC and that there was also some evidence of deactivation of rostral ACC in PTSD as compared with healthy control and trauma-exposed controls, but that there seems to be no differences in the hippocampus or dACC between these groups (Hughes & Shin, 2011; Sartory et al., 2013).

Across the literature to date, trauma-related and general threat stimuli reliably produce higher amygdala activation in PTSD patients compared with nontrauma and trauma controls (Hughes & Shin, 2011). Moreover, the degree of amygdala activity is related to PTSD symptom severity and self-reported anxiety, and amygdala activation is higher in PTSD than nontrauma and trauma control groups during threat provocation tasks (e.g., Britton et al., 2005; Negreira & Abdallah, 2019).

Given the role of fear learning in PTSD and extinction learning in PE, an understanding of how these processes work, both in PTSD and healthy controls, is critical to an understanding of how PE promotes recovery at the level of brain function and structure. Research to date supports a critical role for fear learning neurocircuitry in the development and effective treatment of PTSD. Specifically, the most consistent results indicate that patients with PTSD compared with healthy controls show deficits in recall of extinction learning (Milad et al., 2009). *Extinction learning* occurs when an organism (person) who has paired a stimulus with a negative or feared outcome encounters that stimulus repeatedly without a feared outcome. When this happens, the organism starts to associate that stimulus less with fear and more with safety and, consequently, reacts with less fear. When the organism later encounters that stimulus, if extinction learning is retained, the organism will have the lower fear reaction. If the extinction learning is not retained, the organism may have more fear reaction or even have the original fear reaction (called *spontaneous recovery*). As previously mentioned, PTSD is most consistently associated with deficits in extinction retention, such that a person with PTSD is more likely to have a return of fear in a trauma-related situation even if they have encountered that situation repeatedly without a negative or feared outcome. It is important to note here that fear learning and extinction learning can be context dependent. This may also impact whether fear reactions continue over time. This deficit in extinction recall is associated with hyperactive amygdala, insula, and dACC (Garfinkel et al., 2014; Milad et al., 2009). Extinction learning and retention are key processes involved in exposure-based treatments, such as PE. Indeed, a key target of PE is reduction of fear and negative emotional reactions in response to trauma stimuli. Finding ways to enhance extinction learning and generalize retention is considered a promising direction to enhance the efficiency and efficacy of PE. In addition, PTSD patients show evidence of hypoactive hippocampus (Admon et al., 2013) and medial prefrontal cortal (mPFC; Garfinkel et al., 2014) as compared with healthy controls. Both hippocampus and mPFC are involved in extinction learning and retention (see additional details below; Milad et al., 2009). In their review of neuroimaging of PTSD, Hughes and Shin also concluded that increased activation of dACC in PTSD compared with trauma-exposed controls is related to PTSD severity (Hughes & Shin, 2011). Hughes and Shin qualified this conclusion in their review, because it may be due to familial risk since the one twin study that examined it found this pattern of activation in PTSD patients and in their PTSD-unaffected co-twins (Hughes & Shin, 2011; Pitman et al., 2006).

When focusing on emotion regulation, neuroimaging studies have found low mPFC volume in PTSD patients compared with normal controls (Meng et al., 2016). Further, the magnitude of volume difference is associated with PTSD severity (Meng et al., 2016). Finally, Thomaes et al. (2014) showed improvement in mPFC function following effective PTSD treatment. Together, these findings provide compelling support for the role of mPFC in PTSD development and treatment response, with the capacity for emotion regulation as a potential behavioral indicator.

The hippocampus plays the key role in contextual learning, including fear learning and extinction processes that are highly relevant to the development and treatment of PTSD (Milad et al., 2009). Indeed, in healthy humans, the ability to respond to stimuli differentially on the basis of situational context appears to reside in the hippocampus. The research findings on hippocampal response in PTSD have been mixed, potentially due to variations in task specifications related to context. Specifically, for fear learning and extinction paradigms, if the context of exposure to the aversive stimulus is not accounted for or attended to, resulting outcomes may differ for PTSD patients and healthy controls. From extensive laboratory research on fear learning and extinction, we know that when the fear stimulus is coded in the brain during fear learning it includes information on context— the what, where, and how associated with the threat (Shechner et al., 2014). Similarly, when extinction learning occurs, the context associated with the fear stimulus also changes, and these changes may be broad (as when the extinction generalizes across a wide range of contexts) or specific (as when the extinction is restricted to a much smaller range of context or possibly just to the extinction learning context). The process of contextualization is key in both fear learning (when the person is exposed to threat they may say everything is dangerous or only a few key places and people are dangerous) and extinction (when the person says this specific context is less dangerous but every other one remains dangerous or when they say this situation is safe and therefore think all situations are now safe).

The hippocampus appears to play a key role in these contextual processes (Anagnostaras et al., 2001). In their review, Hughes and Shin (2011) concluded that posttrauma processes that involve the hippocampus, such as decontextualization of fear learning (the organism generalizing the threat across a very wide range of stimuli), led to more frequent activation of threat response in PTSD compared with healthy controls, and appeared to impact overgeneralization of fear learning through neurotoxic effects on the hippocampus. From emotional processing theory that is the basis of PE, providing a new context for the trauma memory is a key target for the intervention. This occurs as the patient approaches the memory and thinks about what it means for them at the time of the trauma and now, as well as in in vivo exposures where the patient learns previously feared or avoided situations are relatively safe. Importantly, some research supports that hippocampal differences may be present prior to trauma exposure, with the posttrauma processes described above then exacerbating a preexisting risk factor for PTSD. Specifically, Pitman et al. (2006) found smaller hippocampal volume in those with PTSD and their cotwins without PTSD. As such, these processes may represent a risk factor for the development of PTSD if exposed to trauma or to a process that differentiates after trauma, or possibly both impacts occur (risk factor starts the differentiation and then it becomes further differentiated over time following trauma).

With the rise of functional connectivity studies, new theoretical models are gaining use and utility. The triple network model as applied in PTSD proposes that alterations in the central executive, salience, and default mode networks contribute to PTSD (Negreira & Abdallah, 2019; Patel et al., 2012). The *central executive network* (CEN) is critical in verbal learning and executive function (e.g., planning and inhibiting response). The *salience network* (SN) is crucial to stimulus detection and to directing action to the most important environmental stimuli. The *default mode network* (DMN) is involved in processes that connect to the self, such as social cognition, autobiographical memory, and self-referential processing (Lanius et al., 2015). Specifically, deficits in the CEN, including underutilization of dorsolateral prefrontal cortex (dlPFC) and lateral areas of the parietal lobe and overutilization of the precuneus have been found related to PTSD compared with healthy controls (Patel et al., 2012). The salience network (anterior insula and dACC) is overactivated and the default mode network (posterior cingulate cortex, posterior inferior parietal lobule, and left hippocampal gyrus) is underactivated in PTSD (Patel et al., 2012). PTSD is associated with greater within-salience network connectivity (Abdallah et al., 2019), lower within-DMN connectivity (Akiki et al., 2018; Lazarov et al., 2017), and greater desegregation or cross-network SN-DMN connectivity (V. M. Brown et al., 2014; Sripada et al., 2012). A recent meta-analysis of resting state studies also partially supports this model (T. Wang et al., 2016).

What Does This Mean for PE?

Research using neuroimaging to examine brain processes that are relevant to treatment and over the course of treatment has truly taken off over the past 5 years. Even with exciting new findings as described below, the expense and variability inherent in the use of imaging for clinical care makes it still aspirational as a tool for individual patient treatment planning. S. A. M. Rauch and Liberzon (2016) summarized the literature and provided a heuristic model for the neural mechanisms of PTSD and change with treatment, with two possible paths for treatment response. The first path involves down-regulation of activity in the brain regions involved in emotion generation, such as the amygdala, dACC, and insula. This path would include many of the changes involved in extinction learning and retention of extinction learning. The second path involves negative emotion regulation through reducing the amplitude and duration of reactivity to negative stimuli. This path may be more related to improvements in affect tolerance. Of note, for most of the research reviewed and conducted to date, it is unclear whether the differences found in brain function and structure in PTSD are a reflection of biological differences that preexist trauma exposure and convey risk for PTSD development or whether these differences occur following trauma exposure as PTSD develops. Consistent with the above, Thomaes et al.'s (2014) review of neuroimaging concluded that effective psychotherapy for PTSD was related to decreased amygdala activation and increased prefrontal, dorsal anterior cingulate, and hippocampal activations possibly related to extinction learning and retention. To take this another step, regardless of whether these differences preexist trauma or occur following trauma, it is also unclear whether the differences observed can "normalize" or partially return to function that is more similar to healthy control populations and whether that may be related to return to normal function. Indeed, it is entirely possible that instead of trying to "normalize" function to what occurs in healthy controls, effective recovery may be possible through the activation of new compensatory mechanisms.

One of the first notable studies examining imaging as it relates to PE treatment response showed that greater activation of the ventral ACC and mPFC during nonconscious threat processing was related to less reduction in PTSD severity following a cognitive behavioral therapy that included imaginal and in vivo exposure (Bryant, Felmingham, et al., 2008). The study task involved masked presentation of emotional faces (threat and nonthreat) at a rate that could not be detected consciously in order to examine the initial response to such emotional stimuli. This study also found that greater activation of the dACC and less activation of the amygdala during nonconscious threat processing was related to larger reduction of PTSD severity during treatment (Bryant, Felmingham, et al., 2008). Such processes may reflect differences in initial affect tolerance that is part of inhibitory learning, and they may suggest an individual difference variable such that people who are better able to tolerate negative affect can accomplish the tasks required in trauma-focused therapy more fully and thus are more able to achieve an effective dose of exposure to reduce the symptoms of PTSD. Additional research is necessary to determine if this is the case.

Zhu et al. (2018) found increased functional connectivity between the amygdala, hippocampus, and prefrontal regions following PE in patients with PTSD but no changes in trauma-exposed healthy controls over the same time period. These changes may reflect improvements with fear inhibition and extinction learning that occur in PE (Stojek et al., 2018). Additional research examining changes with treatment is needed.

Building on these findings, Charquero-Ballester et al. (2020) used a new data-driven approach to define the brain networks that are activated during a trauma provocation task (personal trauma script) and found that people with PTSD activate two DMN subnetworks for less time than trauma controls and that time in salience network during trauma reminders correlated to PTSD severity (Charquero-Ballester et al., 2020). This study also showed that following effective treatment using the Ehlers model of cognitive therapy for PTSD that includes significant discussion of the trauma memory and reminders, the difference between PTSD patients and trauma controls were no longer apparent posttreatment, suggesting a normalization of function resulting from treatment (Charquero-Ballester et al., 2020).

Several studies have recently isolated baseline predictors of response to psychotherapy, including PE. In an examination to determine whether patients who would respond to exposure-based treatment (provided in standard care with either EMDR or trauma-focused cognitive behavioral therapy [CBT] could be identified at baseline), Zhutovksy et al. (2019) found the treatment responder and nonresponder groups differed in a resting state network centered on the bilateral superior frontal gyrus and that differences in a network centered on the presupplementary motor area separated responders and nonresponders at the individual level.

In a randomized controlled trial examining patients receiving PE across time using fMRI, Fonzo et al. (2017) found that patients who had larger reductions in PTSD symptoms during PE showed (a) greater dorsal prefrontal activation (dACC, anterior insula, and dlPFC) and less left amygdala activation during emotional reactivity, (b) better inhibition of the left amygdala induced by transcranial magnetic stimulation (TMS) over the right dlPFC, and (c) greater ventromedial prefrontal/ventral striatal activation during emotional conflict regulation. The authors concluded that the ability to benefit from PE may be restricted by the patient's baseline capacity for prefrontal control over amygdala activation to threat and by the ability to reduce interference from environmental emotional cues.

With an innovative approach taking advantage of the complexity of imaging data, Etkin et al. (2019) identified a combined phenotype linked to greater symptom reduction in response to PE. Specifically, using baseline functional connectivity and verbal memory task data, patients showing aberrant functional connectivity in the ventral attention network combined with impaired verbal memory on a word list learning task showed less response to PE. Although promising, it is unclear whether this finding will replicate and demonstrate the sensitivity and specificity necessary to be used for individual-patient-level treatment planning. Further, it remains unknown whether these findings are specific to PTSD or specific to PE as opposed to a general psychotherapy marker. Additional research is needed and ongoing. Of note, Etkin et al. (2019) took the bold step to establish a more clinically efficient imaging protocol with EEG to mirror the fMRI findings to broaden the possible clinical utility of these markers.

When looking for predictors of response to therapy and medication treatment for PTSD, S. A. M. Rauch et al. (2019) conducted a treatment outcome and mechanisms study comparing three conditions: (a) PE plus placebo, (b) PE plus sertraline, and (c) sertraline plus enhanced medication management.

Duval et al. (2020) presented results from examination of emotion processing and regulation in a task that examined implicit emotion processing, attention modulation of emotion, and appraisal of emotion from the S. A. M. Rauch et al. (2019) study. Specifically, at pretreatment they found that greater activation in the anterior insula and prefrontal cortex and increased connectivity between the dlPFC and superior parietal cortex and amygdala were related to superior treatment outcomes regardless of treatment group. Thus, enhanced connectivity within attention control regions was associated with symptom improvement. Further, patients who begin treatment with better connectivity between executive control networks and emotional processing networks derive more treatment benefit (Duval et al., 2020). When examining an emotional faces task and another emotion regulation task in this same clinical trial, Joshi et al. (2020) found that less dorsomedial prefrontal cortex (dmPFC) activation at baseline during reappraisal of negative emotions was associated with larger reductions in PTSD across the three treatment groups. Thus, these changes may be related to mechanisms of general treatment response that are not specific to PE or medication. Replication and extension to larger samples is needed.

CONCLUSION

Although a good amount of promising research has been conducted to date, the sum of the evidence has not yet provided clarity and specificity about the processes involved in the development of PTSD in the brain, which biomarkers predict treatment response, or what therapeutic recovery looks like in the brain. Continued examination and extension of previous studies to additional treatment samples is needed in order to move the field forward in our understanding, and even more studies are needed to apply the findings from imaging research to individual-patient-level decision making for diagnosis and treatment (Prasad et al., 2019).

5
ELECTROENCEPHALOGRAPHY

In this chapter, we summarize research using electroencephalogram (EEG) as it informs the development and effective treatment of posttraumatic stress disorder (PTSD). To date, the research in this area has been sparse and often not replicated. We also discuss recent advances in EEG, such as the more recently used methods of evoked potentials and new modeling techniques, combined with the addition of more recording channels allowing for higher resolution, more precise localization of activity, and imaging of deeper brain processes than ever before. These advances have led many imaging researchers to look back at how functional magnetic resonance imaging (fMRI) findings may present in EEG given the comparative advantages of EEG for portability and cost. We conclude this chapter with a discussion of the necessary research steps to extend previous fMRI findings to this new tool.

METHODS FOR SCIENTIFIC DISCOVERY

EEG is a method of recording brain electrical potentials over time from sensors on the scalp during either resting state (where a subject/person is not instructed in any specific activity or direction but simply monitored over time)

https://doi.org/10.1037/0000242-005
Retraining the Brain: Applied Neuroscience in Exposure Therapy for PTSD,
by S. A. M. Rauch and C. P. McLean

or during a specific task (targeting specific brain processes or functions, such as a memory task or emotion perception or regulation task, etc.). The subject has a cap with electrodes placed on the head that are connected to a recording device. The *electrical potentials* are then extracted in the frequency, time domain, or both. Data transformations (beyond the scope of this chapter) are then used to establish the power spectrum of a signal usually within a frequency band (Butt et al., 2019). *Peak frequency* (the highest amplitude within a given band per individual) is often used as a measure of locality of brain activity (Butt et al., 2019). *Connectivity* (amplitude or power correlations between electrodes) is commonly examined as a way to look at the interconnections of processes across different brain regions (Butt et al., 2019). Recent advances have allowed EEG caps to have more electrodes than ever before and even have wireless recording rather than the many wires of typical EEG. With additional electrodes (up to 128 is common for research applications, although 19 is typical for standard clinical use) and better modeling methodology, neuroscientists are now able to more precisely locate brain activity, and they can even provide suggestions of deeper brain activity, compared with what was possible even 10 years ago.

Over the many years that EEGs have been in use, the collection and processing of the data obtained has taken many forms. Although these calculations are complex and beyond the focus of the current chapter, a high-level understanding of where they arise is helpful. Current practice for examination of PTSD and the processes relevant to the treatment of PTSD falls into two common techniques: (a) *event-related potentials* (ERPs; including specific methods such as mismatch negativity [MMNs] and late positive potentials [LPPs] that are described later) and (b) *connectivity analysis* (similar to how this term is used in fMRI).

Event-Related Potentials

EEG data are often analyzed with reference to a specific stimulus or task-related event, such as an aversive or a happy picture that is viewed or a blast of loud sound. Most paradigms include multiple presentations of various types of stimuli, with some as target stimuli and some as comparison stimuli. When these responses are averaged over multiple presentations over time, the *noise* (or variance in the electrical signal that is due to causes other than activation from the stimulus) that contaminates a single activation is reduced. The investigators are then better able to isolate the response that is related to that specific stimulus more precisely. These averages are called ERPs. ERPs are usually examined with respect to differences in amplitude or latency (time from stimulus onset to peak amplitude), or both, across task conditions (e.g., threat vs. nonthreat) or groups of patients (e.g., PTSD vs. trauma controls). ERPs are often referred to as components such as *P200* (P2; a positive peak that occurs at roughly 200 ms) or *N400* (a negative nadir that occurs at roughly 400 ms). Each component is thought to relate to certain brain processes, such as attention, memory consolidation, and so on (Butt et al., 2019). See Table 5.1 for a summary of the most common ERP components examined in PTSD research.

TABLE 5.1. Event-Related Potentials (ERPs) Examined in PTSD Research

ERP name	Timing in milliseconds (ms)	Description
P200 (or P2)	Peak at about 200 ms	Stimulus detection, selective attention and short-term memory retrieval[a]
P300 (or P3)	Peak at about 300 ms	Elicited in response to an attended target prior to response generation; related to memory consolidation of stimulus evaluation, active stimuli discrimination and motivational contextual salience[a]
N170	Nadir at about 170 ms	Response activated specifically based on face stimuli[a]
N200	Nadir at about 200 ms	Detects deviant stimuli while attending to standard stimuli[a]
N400 (or N4)	Nadir at about 400 ms	Linked to meaning processing[b]
Contingent negative variation (CNV)	Nadir at about 600 ms after cue onset	Related to anticipatory reactions to an expected stimulus and associated with working memory and motor/perceptual timing[a]
Error-related negativity (ERN)	Nadir at about 50–150 ms following error	Related to commission of an error in a target task[c]
Mismatch negativity (MMN)	Nadir at about 120 ms	Sensory memory system and preattentive processing[a]
Late positive potential (LPP)	Peak at between 400 and 1000 ms	Related to evaluation of emotional content[a]

[a]As summarized in Butt et al. (2019). [b]As summarized in Kutas and Federmeier (2011). [c]As summarized in Wessel (2012).

EEG Band Power

Another common analytic technique used in EEG involves breaking the signals up into specific bands of frequencies (typically alpha, beta, delta, gamma, and theta; Newson & Thiagarajan, 2019). *Alpha band* is the most commonly reported within the PTSD literature. Specifics of how these calculations are made are beyond the scope of this chapter, but *absolute power* refers to a summation of a specific band frequency over a time period, whereas *relative power* typically refers to activation in a time period in one band in comparison with the power across all bands together. See Newson and Thiagarajan (2019) for a thorough review of processing techniques. These bands are related to different types of brain activity, such as attentional and memory processes. Alpha band power is the most studied within PTSD at present. In addition to band power, *asymmetry* is another tool used to examine EEG signals. This commonly involves comparison of power within a specific band in the left hemisphere and with the same right hemisphere power band (Sun et al., 2017). Asymmetry is often related to different disorders (e.g., PTSD, depression, attention-deficit/hyperactivity disorder [ADHD]) and is thought to reflect problematic cognitive, memory, or emotional processing.

Connectivity

Although activation in specific areas is important, fMRI research using connectivity analysis has demonstrated the importance of the impact of changes in activation and deactivation in one area as it relates to functioning in other areas of the brain. With more precise EEG systems in use today and advances in signal modeling, connectivity analysis of EEG now allows investigators to examine how specific activity in one area may relate to activity in another area. Use of connectivity analysis in EEG is becoming more common and promises to increase the utility of EEG as a clinical and research tool.

Tasks

The descriptions in Table 5.1 relate to general interpretations of ERPs, but it is important to note that the timing and type of reactions are highly dependent on the stimulus or task presentation. Common paradigms used in EEG vary widely on the basis of what specific processes are under investigation. Whereas many studies use resting state, where the subject is simply orienting to a stimulus while the recordings are collected, other studies have specific tasks that are used to probe for types of activity, such as emotion processing, error processing, and the like. Tasks often used to compare PTSD and trauma-exposed, or healthy controls, include the Stroop task or emotional Stroop task (Scarpina & Tagini, 2017), dot-probe, flanker task, go/no-go, and so forth. The *Stroop task* presents words in word consistent or inconsistent color (e.g., the word "black" in a green font or a black font). The subject is asked to either say the word or say the color of the word, with the inconsistent trials requiring more time because of the interference that occurs. The *emotional Stroop task* uses emotion words consistent with an emotional state that is of interest (e.g., sad words for examination of depression; trauma words for PTSD) to see if the patient responds faster or slower to specific emotionally valanced words. Dot-probe paradigms place a person in front of a screen staring at a fixation point while target and nontarget stimuli are presented on either side of the fixation for varying amounts of time. A dot then appears on one side or the other. The person is asked to respond as quickly as possible with which side the dot appeared. This procedure can assess many perceptual biases depending on which probes are presented (emotional, trauma specific, etc.) and for how long (conscious vs. preconscious; MacLeod et al., 1986). *Flanker tasks* are response inhibition tasks designed to test how well a person can inhibit a response based on context (Eriksen & Eriksen, 1974), for instance, only hitting the button when there are two right-pointing arrows followed by a left-pointing arrow. *Go/no-go tasks* similarly assess inhibitory control (Gomez et al., 2007). Additional review of the many different potential probe tasks is beyond the limits of this chapter, but task descriptions are presented below to ease interpretation.

WHAT DOES THIS MEAN FOR PTSD?

In their comprehensive review of EEG findings to date, Butt et al. (2019) concluded that greater right than left parietal asymmetry in the alpha band power is higher in PTSD compared with trauma controls and healthy controls. They also concluded that the magnitude of this asymmetry is associated with greater physiological arousal, which in turn may impair the ability to filter out environmental distractors. This may be a marker of "decontextualized" emotional activation or generalization, in which patients with PTSD are activated across contexts and others are activated only in the context paired with previous danger. In addition, Butt et al. concluded that with regard to ERPs, increased frontocentral responses (including contingent negative variation [CNV], mismatch negativity [MMN], and P300 amplitudes) to task-relevant distractors and reduced parietal responses to task-relevant target stimuli also support a decontextualized response in PTSD. For instance, in one of the studies reviewed,

Bangel et al. (2017) found that patients with PTSD showed enhanced MMN and stronger suppression of upper alpha activity after deviant compared with standard tones when compared with trauma-exposed controls. In addition, the magnitude of this suppression was related to spatial working memory impairment. Similarly, in a review examining posttraumatic stress symptom severity, Lobo et al. (2015) concluded that posttraumatic stress severity is most consistently related to P200 and P300 ERP and alpha rhythm alterations. These markers suggested problems with attention processes that may have significant impact on memory and function.

Research focusing on the development of PTSD following trauma has found that problems with processing emotionally valanced information is linked with PTSD risk. Fitzgerald et al. (2018) found that deficiencies in emotion reappraisal (less change in LPPs) predicted more PTSD symptoms over time in a sample of trauma-exposed combat veterans. More specifically, this means that combat veterans who were less able to reevaluate emotional stimuli in a way to reduce their negative emotional reactions to the stimuli maintained more PTSD symptoms over time. In addition, reduction in avoidance symptoms over time was associated with a greater reduction in neural response to reappraisal over time. Using a flanker task to examine error-related negativity (ERN) risk profiles (i.e., patterns that predict specific outcomes such as PTSD) for combat veterans, Khan et al. (2018) found that greater combat exposure, and not PTSD diagnosis, had enhanced ERNs, even after adjusting for PTSD and general anxiety.

One of the key symptoms of PTSD is sleep disturbance, including both nightmares (PTSD intrusive cluster) and other sleep disturbance (PTSD hypervigilance cluster; American Psychiatric Association, 2013). Academic research and debates are ongoing about whether sleep disturbance in PTSD is a secondary or core feature (Spoormaker & Montgomery, 2008). One of the key tools of sleep medicine is a sleep study that typically includes EEG (and other recordings) over the course of a night or several nights of sleep. Modarres et al. (2019) examined EEG across sleep and wake states to determine whether PTSD-specific predictive biomarkers can be extracted. Using novel coherence markers that combined information gathered in both sleep and wake states, they found a diagnostic marker that distinguishes PTSD from non-PTSD in veterans with 83% accuracy and a PTSD severity marker that was reliable as well. These sleep measures provide a fertile ground to further explore for PTSD biomarkers, as this type of EEG becomes more portable and avoids any patient-related reporting bias (Modarres et al., 2019). Although encouraging, these findings require replication and extension to larger samples before clinical use is warranted.

Given high rates of PTSD combined with traumatic brain injury (TBI), many have worked to find ways to distinguish these injuries on the basis of imaging and EEG. In a study of veterans ($N = 147$; 40 with PTSD and 115 with mild TBI [mTBI]; not mutually exclusive groups), Franke et al. (2016) found that PTSD was associated with decreases in low frequency power, especially in the right temporoparietal region, whereas mTBI was associated with increases in low frequency power, especially in the prefrontal and right temporal regions. As noted above, if replicated, this finding would also provide key clinical differential diagnostic information to guide clinical care on who may benefit from cognitive rehabilitation in addition to PTSD treatment.

Another common comorbidity with PTSD is depression. Rates of co-occurrence range from about 32% to as high as 60% in treatment-seeking samples (Knowles et al., 2019; Wisco et al., 2014). S.-H. Lee et al. (2014) found EEG activation patterns that discriminated depression severity from PTSD severity. They also found that decreased resting state functional connectivity discriminated PTSD from healthy controls and that the degree of this reduction was correlated with PTSD severity. As such, this differential EEG can also inform treatment planning.

WHAT DOES THIS MEAN FOR PE?

Few studies to date have used EEG across treatment to examine change in brain function related to treatment response. One study focused on PE and found that after successful PE, right hemisphere EEG activation was reduced and the magnitude of reduction was associated with reduction in PTSD over treatment (Rabe et al., 2008). These changes have been suggested to reflect extinction learning, with resulting reduced fear expression following PE.

As noted in Chapter 4 on imaging results, several changes in brain structure and function have been correlated with PTSD treatment change, and efforts to approximate and measure those changes through less invasive EEG have been pursued by many. In their work to identify baseline biomarkers of treatment response, Etkin et al. (2019) used EEG combined with transcranial magnetic stimulation (TMS) to examine visual attention network connectivity and verbal memory, using a very brief verbal memory delayed-recall task. They found that patients who showed low within-ventral attention network (VAN) connectivity and impaired verbal memory experienced minimal recovery following PE. The percentage of patients out of the full PTSD treatment sample who met these criteria was not reported. These findings need to be replicated and extended to larger samples and examination of sensitivity and specificity of the prediction is required. If the results replicate, this biomarker could be used at baseline to identify patients who will benefit from PE and those who may need a different treatment approach (either augmentation of PE, additional medication, or an alternate treatment approach, such as yoga, etc.). Relatedly, in a small pilot study, PTSD patients with working memory deficits (who completed computerized working memory training with direct current stimulation) showed improvements on a cognitive and emotional performance measure that coincided with pre- to posttreatment change in P300 ERP in response to novelty (Saunders et al., 2015). Additional work needs to determine whether these findings replicate in other (larger) samples and whether this pattern is unique to PTSD or exists in other disorders as well. In addition, examination of the prevalence of working memory deficits as defined in Saunders et al. (2015) or Etkin et al. (2019) among PTSD treatment–seeking patients is key. Work will also be needed to determine if working memory training is its own stand-alone treatment option or an augmentation for PE or other psychotherapies for PTSD patients identified at baseline as unlikely to respond or to respond more slowly. Butt et al. (2019) suggested that given the attentional difficulties associated with PTSD, providing specific cognitive attentional training prior to PE, either for all patients or only those identified as "at risk" of slower response, may speed response or increase efficacy directly.

CONCLUSION

These advances have led many imaging researchers to look back at how fMRI findings may present in EEG given the comparative advantages of EEG for portability and cost. Indeed, many see EEG as a more feasible tool for use in clinical assessment and treatment than fMRI. EEG is less invasive, as the patient can sit with a cap on outside of a magnet or other imaging machine. With the availability of portable EEGs and even wireless models, this allows for mobility during measurement. EEG provides better temporal resolution. For activations that are tied to stimulus and response, such as fear learning and extinction, this is better able to see more precise changes.

To translate what we know about PTSD and brain function into clinical care, many have begun to examine fMRI and EEG simultaneously to use potential correlates of identified fMRI signatures of PTSD and treatment response that can be examined using EEG in clinical care. Yuan et al. (2018) used the methodology of microstates and found EEG microstates that correlated with dorsal default mode network and salience network alterations in PTSD as compared with healthy controls, and these were related to PTSD severity as well.

In conclusion, EEG is a long-standing and flexible tool for examining emotional and cognitive function. Recent advances provide an opportunity for EEG to bridge the gap between what we have learned from brain imaging research and clinical research and practice. Continued work is necessary to establish EEG markers of brain processes that can be used in clinical settings as diagnostic and prognostic biomarkers of PTSD and its responses to treatment. In the future, such EEG markers may provide a real-time, cost-effective, and less burdensome tool for use in standard clinical practice.

6 PSYCHOPHYSIOLOGY

In this chapter, we summarize the current methods and recent advances of psychophysiological exploration on posttraumatic stress disorder (PTSD) and prolonged exposure (PE). We examine potential diagnostic and prognostic biomarkers of PTSD and treatment response and then discuss how new mobile technologies are making psychophysiological monitoring more user friendly for PE patients and providers. We conclude with how these tools can continue to improve research methods and patient care through real-time monitoring that allows for responsive changes in emotional engagement to optimize exposures and predict those who may be the most responsive to treatment.

METHODS FOR SCIENTIFIC DISCOVERY

Psychophysiological recording includes assessment and collection of information from all components of human physiology as it applies to psychological processes. Although a comprehensive review of psychophysiological research on PTSD is beyond the scope of this book, this chapter focuses on the most promising and consistent findings within specific areas of PTSD (i.e., fear learning and extinction, fear potentiated startle [FPS], and script-driven imagery)

https://doi.org/10.1037/0000242-006
Retraining the Brain: Applied Neuroscience in Exposure Therapy for PTSD,
by S. A. M. Rauch and C. P. McLean

and as applied to PE. Psychophysiological responses in PTSD have been examined since the diagnosis was first developed to operationalize what identifies PTSD as opposed to "normal" posttrauma reactions and to distinguish what may predict future problems in function following trauma. In addition, physiological reactions are included as symptoms of PTSD. Specifically, physiological reactivity to trauma reminders and exaggerated startle response are both symptoms of PTSD. Because the field of psychopathology research defines observable behaviors and neurobiological measures that can be uniformly and objectively collected and examined through Research Doman Criteria (RDoC) and other systems, it may provide a flexible, portable, and real-time tool for examination of PTSD diagnostic and prognostic phenomena (Norrholm et al., 2015). Full explanation of RDoC applied to PTSD is beyond the scope of this book, but interested readers are referred to Schmidt and Vermetten (2017) as well as the National Institute of Mental Health (NIMH) RDoC website (https://www.nimh.nih.gov/research/research-funded-by-nimh/rdoc/index.shtml) for detailed information.

Psychophysiology can be an excellent tool, but it also has notable limitations. First, ambulatory monitoring is often not possible or not accurate for most psychophysiological measures; they are only feasible within a lab. Additionally, the measures require significant expertise and time to score and examine, making real-time use difficult or impossible. Outstanding advances have been made recently to provide more automated scoring and reliable ambulatory equipment, such as eSense (Hinrichs et al., 2017), but additional advances are needed. In addition, populations with higher trauma load and chronic stress, such as Black, Indigenous, and people of color, may respond to psychophysiological measures differently than White populations, leading to misinterpretations of their data or variability when studied if not carefully and specifically examined (Kredlow et al., 2017). Additional work on the influence of individual differences (e.g., race, gender, ethnicity, trauma exposure, etc.) in psychophysiological expression is needed.

WHAT DOES THIS MEAN FOR PTSD?

In a seminal meta-analysis of psychophysiological studies in PTSD, Pole (2007) concluded that PTSD patients showed increased baseline heart rate (HR) and skin conductance and increased startle response (as measured using eyeblink, HR, and skin conductance) compared with combat-exposed controls. In addition, PTSD patients showed slower skin conductance habituation compared with combat-exposed controls. Other research has focused more specifically on high frequency heart rate variability (HRV, the interval between heart beats), controlling for respiration rate, and found that veterans with PTSD have lower HRV than combat controls without PTSD (Wahbeh & Oken, 2013). This is thought to reflect increased sympathetic nervous system dominance but may also be a sign of decontextualization of fear.

Respiratory sinus arrythmia (RSA) is the naturally occurring variation in HR that occurs across the breathing cycle. High RSA (cardiac vagal control) is described as a sign of healthy parasympathetic nervous activity, where the system is responding adaptively to internal and external stimuli. Campbell et al. (2019) used meta-analysis to examine RSA in PTSD across all relevant human studies and found a small but significant relationship between RSA and PTSD that increased with age, with lower RSA among those with PTSD than those without PTSD. As research has progressed, it has become better established that PTSD and trauma control population RSA differences are more robust in response to trauma-specific cues and often not apparent to general negative stimuli (Pineles et al., 2013).

Fear Learning and Extinction

Psychophysiological methods are often used to examine how fear is acquired and maintained over time as a window into processes involved in the development and maintenance of PTSD. For an informative review of current learning models and animal and human research as applied to PTSD, see Lissek and van Meurs (2015). Fear learning includes *fear acquisition* (the process of Pavlovian conditioning, where a previously neutral stimulus is associated with fear/negative outcome) and *extinction* (the process of presentation of the stimulus that was paired with the fear/negative outcome without the negative outcome; Lissek & van Meurs, 2015; Norrholm & Jovanovic, 2018). Many years of human and animal research on fear learning and extinction has demonstrated that extinction learning creates a new memory representing safety that competes with the previous fear memory producing inhibition of fear response. Evidence supporting the development of a new safety memory, rather than the modification of the old fear memory, comes from research showing return of fear under certain circumstances—such as in the presence of context cues that raise salience of the fear memory over the extinction memory (Norrholm & Jovanovic, 2018). Previous research supports that PTSD patients show enhanced fear learning compared with combat-exposed controls in skin conductance response to a fear learning (paired with shock) paradigm (Orr et al., 2000). Other studies have also supported this association, including demonstrating overexpression of acquired fear associations in civilian trauma survivors with PTSD as well as attentional bias toward threat (Fani et al., 2012; Norrholm et al., 2011).

In addition, PTSD is associated with overgeneralization of the conditioned fear response. Psychophysiological research using skin conductance and other measures to assess physiological responsiveness to stimuli as they approximate the target conditioned stimulus has shown that people with PTSD are responsive to a wider number of similar stimuli than those without PTSD (Kaczkurkin et al., 2017). This is called a *generalization gradient*, where a larger gradient means that the target response occurs to stimuli that are less like the fear conditioned target. Although this phenomenon has been established in other anxiety disorders and using imaging, additional work is needed to replicate it in PTSD (Kaczkurkin et al., 2017; Lissek et al., 2008, 2010; Lissek & van Meurs, 2015).

Fear extinction deficits are also apparent in PTSD. In a review and summary, Norrholm and Jovanovic (2018) concluded that these deficits were represented in three potential phenotypes: (a) overexpression of acquired fear (as described above), (b) impaired within-session extinction learning, and (c) reduced between-session extinction recall (less maintenance of extinction learning across sessions/time). The degree of fear, or "fear load," during extinction was predictive of intrusive thoughts and physiological reactivity to trauma reminders in PTSD (Norrholm et al., 2015). Of importance, Zuj et al. (2016) found that the extinction learning deficits demonstrated in PTSD compared with trauma controls were moderated by time since waking, with greater deficits later in the day, suggesting that circadian rhythms and their impact on cortisol or general attentional process deficits due to waning energy later in the day may impact fear learning in PTSD. Thus, consideration of time of day for sessions in patients with PTSD may be warranted.

Fear Potentiated Startle

In addition to standard fear conditioning paradigms, PTSD has also been examined using FPS paradigms. This methodology is based on the biological startle response when presented with a sudden specific aversive stimulus (most often an air blast to the larynx or sudden loud noise) and the tendency for such a response to be augmented in a context that is perceived as threatening compared with a perceived safe context. In such studies, the difference between the startle response in these contexts is considered an index of fear load (Jovanovic & Norrholm, 2016). In addition, these FPS paradigms can also be combined with fear conditioning paradigms, with the startle probe serving as an unconditioned stimulus and with other stimuli (most often shapes presented on a screen) then being conditioned as safety or fear cues depending on study design. Studies have shown that PTSD is related to increased FPS compared with trauma controls and that the amount of increase in FPS is related to the severity of PTSD (Orcutt et al., 2017). In addition, level of subthreshold PTSD symptom severity was related to elevated HR and to startle response to danger cues and poorer skin conductance discrimination between safety and danger (Costanzo et al., 2016).

Finally, fear inhibition is impaired in PTSD compared with trauma controls, meaning that the fear response is more likely to present. This has been examined in FPS paradigms that indicate patients with PTSD show a greater increase in startle response when in the presence of a fear cue (e.g., a combat scene for combat veterans; another fear cue for other types of traumas) compared with a neutral cue than with trauma controls without PTSD, and this has been demonstrated in both combat and civilian trauma groups (Jovanovic et al., 2009, 2010). One study even demonstrated that continued higher elevation of fear during extinction learning is related to level of reported severity of PTSD symptoms in a group of trauma survivors (Orcutt et al., 2017).

Script-Driven Imagery

HR reactivity to a brief personal trauma script has been well established as a specific and sensitive discriminator of PTSD and non-PTSD combat control patients (e.g., Castro-Chapman et al., 2018). The most common version of this paradigm was refined by Orr et al. (1993) and involved presentation of brief (less than 1 minute) pieces of personal trauma scripts. This paradigm showed diagnostic specificity to PTSD and a relationship to symptom severity, with increased HR reactivity related to increased PTSD severity (Castro-Chapman et al., 2018). Others have found personal trauma scripts as a specific discriminator of PTSD in trauma populations, including Vietnam War nurses (Carson et al., 2000), Vietnam War veterans (Keane et al., 1998), and a mixed-trauma sample (Pineles et al., 2013). On the basis of its excellent stability over time and convergent and predictive validity for PTSD with the Clinically Administered PTSD Scale (CAPS), psychophysiological reactivity to script-driven imagery (SDI) has been put forward as an objective measure of PTSD and RDoC construct (Bauer et al., 2013). Psychophysiological reactivity to SDI appears to be one of the most stable potential PTSD biomarkers found to date.

WHAT DOES THIS MEAN FOR PE?

PE is based on emotional processing theory, which asserts that effective treatment of PTSD requires (a) activation of the fear/trauma memory, and (b) incorporation of information inconsistent with the fear/trauma structure.

Given the central role of memory activation to the efficacy of the treatment (via imaginal exposure), psychophysiological assessment has often been used to examine memory activation and emotional engagement with content of the trauma memory, which is thought to be particularly important for successful recovery in PE. In the review below, although we focus on psychophysiological findings, we also include the presentation of subjective reporting of anxious arousal, as measured by subjective units of distress (SUDS), as part of the PE protocol. The results presented here provide a window into whether and how objective markers of arousal and patient perceived arousal may coincide or diverge, because this is relevant to the patient and provider experience of PE.

Fear Activation/Emotional Engagement

Fear activation is often described in both objective (physiological) and subjective (patient report) terms. Physiological fear activation has been examined by looking at HR (most often) as well as skin conductance, eye blink startle magnitude, and electromyogram (the electrical recording of muscular tissue activity). The degree of activation is measured by using the difference between peak recordings on these measures and baseline reactivity. As measured by the SUDS scale (ranging from 0 to 100), subjective fear activation is typically operationalized as peak (or highest) reported fear level minus the baseline level of reported distress.

The hypothesis that fear activation is necessary to achieve successful exposure therapy outcomes has received mixed support in the broader anxiety disorder literature. Early studies of exposure procedures showed that increased physiological arousal prior to flooding (Watson & Marks, 1971) and greater HR reactivity during initial exposure to the feared stimulus as part of systematic desensitization were associated with greater symptom reduction in patients with simple phobias (Borkovec & Sides, 1979; P. J. Lang et al., 1970). Several other studies found inconsistent support for the role of fear activation in exposure therapy outcomes. Among individuals with simple phobia, HR was significantly related to outcomes, but several other indices of fear activation were not (Watson & Marks, 1971). Among patients with panic disorder, Meuret et al. (2012) found that greater initial subjective anxiety was associated with superior outcomes, but that HR, carbon dioxide partial pressure, and respiration rate were not correlated with treatment outcome. Among college students with elevated fear of heights, there was no relationship between HR activation or initial subjective distress and treatment outcome (A. Baker et al., 2010). Among participants with high claustrophobic fears, HR reactivity was not significantly related to outcomes, but higher subjective distress was related to worse post-treatment outcomes (Telch et al., 2004). Although contrary to hypothesis, this was not the only study to find that indices of fear activation were associated with worse outcome (Foa et al., 1983; Kircanski et al., 2012).

Many of the studies examining the effect of physiological and subjective distress during exposure on treatment outcomes in anxiety-related disorders have focused on PTSD samples. As measured by facial expression of fear coded using the Facial Action Coding System, greater fear activation during the first imaginal exposure among women assault survivors with PTSD was associated with greater symptom reduction during PE (Foa, Riggs, et al., 1995). Among Vietnam veterans with PTSD receiving flooding therapy, Pitman et al. (1996) found that initial HR activation was associated with fewer daily intrusive combat memories at posttreatment, whereas subjective distress and other measures of physiological activation (skin conductance and electromyogram) were not associated with any outcomes. Similarly, veterans with PTSD who showed more HR reactivity to trauma-specific cues at baseline showed more change in PTSD with PE (Wangelin & Tuerk, 2015). Further, they also showed more change in HR and skin conductance to trauma cues over treatment. Most recently, Wisco et al. (2016) found that initial HR activation during written exposure therapy for PTSD was associated with more treatment reduction in PTSD.

In contrast to the above psychophysiological findings, subjective distress has not been consistently associated with treatment outcomes. Jaycox et al. (1998) found that those with higher subjective distress had greater improvements in PTSD symptoms during PE than those with lower subjective distress. In contrast, Pitman et al. (1996) found that subjective distress was not associated with any outcomes. Among patients with PTSD categorized as either responders, nonresponders, or treatment dropouts, van Minnen and Hagenaars (2002) found no differences between groups in mean and peak subjective distress during the first imaginal exposure. Similarly, among women with borderline personality disorder and PTSD, subjective distress and ratings of negative emotions were not related to outcomes (Harned et al., 2015). Two PTSD studies also found null findings for the relationships between initial subjective distress (Bluett et al., 2014) and imagery vividness with treatment outcomes following PE (S. A. M. Rauch et al., 2004). In summary, although there are studies showing that initial fear activation is associated with better treatment outcomes, at least on some measures, there are just as many studies that found no relationship between fear activation and outcome. Among anxiety disorders broadly, a minority found a negative relationship between fear activation and outcome. With PTSD, null findings are more common when examining subjective distress than psychophysiological arousal.

WITHIN-SESSION EXTINCTION

Within-session extinction (WSE) refers to the degree to which anxiety or distress decreases during a single extinction session (made up of many trials) or session of exposure therapy (made up of more than one trial/time recalling the target trauma memory). Many clinical and experimental studies have examined the relationship between WSE and treatment outcomes following exposure therapy for anxiety-related conditions. WSE has been measured by examining changes in physiological measures of anxious arousal including HR and skin conductance and subjective distress.

Although it is typical for anxiety to decline from the beginning to the end of an exposure session, the role of WSE as an indicator of emotional processing has not been well supported. Only a small number of studies focusing on subjective distress have found a direct relationship between WSE and treatment outcome. Specifically, WSE in subjective distress was associated with greater improvement among patients with obsessive-compulsive disorder (OCD; Foa et al., 1983) and patients with mixed anxiety disorders (Norton et al., 2011). Among contamination-fearful undergraduates, WSE in subjective distress was associated with lower obsession severity but not compulsion severity or reported distress during a behavioral avoidance task, and WSE in HR was not related to any outcomes (Kircanski et al., 2012).

Indirect evidence that supports the role of WSE has been found in several studies showing that WSE is greater among participants who showed better outcomes, either based on study condition or a post-hoc categorization. This has been found for HR among snake-fearful women (P. J. Lang et al., 1970), for subjective distress among individuals with flying phobia (Beckham et al., 1990), for speech phobic undergraduates (Borkovec & Sides, 1979; Chaplin & Levine, 1981), and for blood-injection fearful participants (Oliver & Page, 2003). Although the results of these studies are consistent with WSE being indicatory of emotional processing, they do not demonstrate that WSE is directly related to outcomes.

In contrast, many more studies have failed to find support for the relationship between WSE and outcomes in the broader anxiety literature. Null results have been found in studies of patients with OCD for HR and subjective distress (Grayson et al., 1982) and for HR, electrodermal activity, and subjective anxiety (Kozak et al., 1988). Similarly, in patients with panic disorder, null findings for WSE were found for electromyopgraphy, galvanic skin response, and HR (Riley et al., 1995) and for cardiorespiratory physiology and subjective distress (Meuret et al., 2012). Nonclinical samples of participants with elevated height fears (A. Baker et al., 2010; A. J. Lang & Craske, 2000), fear of public speaking

(Culver et al., 2012; Tsao & Craske, 2000), and claustrophobic fears (Kamphuis & Telch, 2000; T. Sloan & Telch, 2002) have also all failed to find support for the relationship between WSE, measured in various ways, and exposure outcomes.

Within PTSD studies specifically, the pattern is much the same. Only one study has looked at WSE in psychophysiological measures. Pitman et al. (1996) found that WSE on several physiological and subjective indices of anxiety were not significantly related to outcome, although there was a trend for WSE in HR to correlate with the number of trauma intrusions per day, which was one of several PTSD-related outcomes examined. In terms of WSE in subjective distress, one study of PE augmentation with d-cycloserine (DCS, a medication that provides cognitive enhancement of learning) found that WSE in subjective distress predicted posttreatment outcomes, with no differences between those receiving DCS or placebo (de Kleine et al., 2015). Providing indirect evidence of a WSE-outcome relationship, van Minnen and Hagenaars (2002) found that WSE in subjective distress was greater among PE responders than PE nonresponders, but only for imaginal exposures completed for homework, not those completed during sessions. In contrast, several PTSD studies have found null results for WSE. Jaycox et al. (1998) found that WSE in subjective distress was unrelated to PE outcomes among sexual assault survivors. Harned et al. (2014), found no relationship between within-session changes in subjective distress and exposure outcomes among women with borderline personality disorder and PTSD. Similarly, Sripada and Rauch (2015) found that WSE in subjective distress was unrelated to symptom change and responder status following PE.

In a nonrandomized study, van Minnen and Foa (2006) found that WSE was greater among participants who received 60 minutes of imaginal exposure than those who received 30 minutes, but there were no group differences in treatment outcomes. This finding was replicated in another study showing that WSE was greater following 40 minutes versus 20 minutes of imaginal exposures, but there were no differences in outcome between groups (Nacasch et al., 2015). These latter studies suggest that although longer exposures are associated with greater WSE, this does not impact outcomes. Thus, in general, although some studies have found that WSE relates to outcomes following exposure, at least for some measures, most studies have not.

BETWEEN-SESSION EXTINCTION

Between-session extinction (BSE) refers to the degree to which peak anxiety decreases across extinction sessions (each session made up of several trials) or sessions of exposure therapy (each session made up of more than one trial/

repetition of the target trauma memory). BSE has been measured by examining changes in the same kind of physiological measures as WSE and subjective distress from one exposure session to the next. In general, evidence for a relationship between BSE and exposure therapy outcomes has been found more consistently than for activation or WSE. However, the evidence remains mixed.

Several studies of anxiety-related disorders have found support for the role of BSE on some indices of BSE on some outcomes. Among patients with OCD, Kozak et al. (1988) showed that BSE in HR (but not electrodermal activity) was also linked to lower fear and avoidance (but not rituals), and there was a nonsignificant trend for BSE in subjective distress to link with lower-rated fear and avoidance as well. Among height-fearful participants, A. Baker et al. (2010) found that BSE in subjective distress (but not HR) across two exposure sessions was linked with lower reported distress during a behavioral avoidance task (but not to self-reported fear of heights). Among patients with OCD, Kircanski et al. (2012) found that BSE in HR was linked with lower obsessions and reported distress but not compulsions, whereas BSE in subjective distress was unrelated to outcomes. Also, in OCD, Foa et al. (1983) found that BSE in subjective anxiety was associated with superior outcomes at posttreatment; however, this did not hold at follow-up.

In terms of indirect evidence for the role of BSE on exposure therapy outcomes in anxiety disorders, a study of DCS augmenting virtual reality exposure therapy for acrophobia found that the DCS group had greater BSE in skin conductance and subjective distress and showed greater improvement in acrophobia than the placebo group (Ressler et al., 2004). In participants with claustrophobia fears, T. Sloan and Telch (2002) found that exposure plus guided reappraisal was associated with greater BSE in subjective distress and superior outcomes at posttreatment, but not at follow-up, compared with exposure plus safety-seeking behavior or exposure alone. In blood-injection fearful participants, Oliver and Page (2003) found that distraction during exposure was linked with greater BSE in subjective distress and superior outcomes at posttreatment and follow-up relative to focusing on the phobic stimuli or standard exposure. In contrast, Telch et al. (2004) found that distraction during exposure led to less BSE in subjective distress and worse outcomes than threat-focused attention or a neutral control group among claustrophobic individuals.

There are also several studies of anxiety disorders that have found no support for the relationship between BSE and exposure outcomes. Meuret et al. (2012) found that BSE in physiological and subjective distress was unrelated to panic disorder treatment outcomes. Similarly, Riley et al. (1995) found that BSE of physiological distress measures was unrelated to responder status in panic disorder patients. Analogue studies by Craske and colleagues (many of which used very short exposure protocols) found similar null results among individuals with spider fears (Rowe & Craske, 1998), public speaking anxiety (Tsao & Craske, 2000), and fears of heights (A. J. Lang & Craske, 2000), with similar findings from Chaplin and Levine (1981) for public speaking anxiety.

Again, the pattern for PTSD is like that seen in the broader anxiety-related disorder literature. There are several studies that found a relationship between BSE and exposure therapy outcomes in PTSD, all of which focus on subjective distress. One exception is the study by Pitman et al. (1996), in which there was a nonsignificant trend for BSE in HR to correlate with the number of intrusions per day. S. A. M. Rauch et al. (2004) observed that greater BSE in subjective distress over the course of six imaginal exposure sessions was associated with more reduction in PTSD symptoms at posttreatment. In contrast to the null findings on WSE, van Minnen and Foa (2006) found that BSE was significantly related to PTSD symptoms at posttreatment among participants with PTSD, regardless of whether they received sessions with 60 or 30 minutes of imaginal exposure. Also, in contrast to null WSE findings, Sripada and Rauch (2015) noted that BSE in subjective distress was related to both symptom change and treatment responder status in participants receiving PE for PTSD. Finally, de Kleine et al. (2015) found that BSE in subjective distress predicted posttreatment outcomes for those receiving PE plus DCS or placebo.

Many PTSD studies also provide indirect support for an association between BSE and exposure outcomes with almost all focusing on subjective distress. Jaycox et al. (1998) found that change during PE fit one of three patterns: (a) high initial fear activation and gradual BSE, (b) high fear activation and no BSE, or (c) moderate fear activation and no BSE; outcomes were superior in the first group. This indicates that BSE in subjective distress, or perhaps the combination of BSE and activation, are common among those with good PE outcomes. BSE in subjective distress was greater among PE responders in a study by van Minnen and Hagenaars (2002), which examined BSE only between the first two exposure sessions. Similarly, BSE significantly predicted PTSD diagnostic and remitter status at posttreatment in a small open trial (Harned et al., 2015). Nacasch et al. (2015) found that, although BSE was greater for those who received 40 versus 20 minutes of imaginal exposure, the groups did not differ on PTSD outcome; however, they also observed that greater BSE was linked with reduction in PTSD symptoms in the full sample. Null results for BSE were found in a large study by Bluett et al. (2014) showing that only 35% of participants who exhibited a reliable change in distress (i.e., reliable BSE) had lower PTSD severity at posttreatment compared with those who did not show reliable BSE. To further complicate, as measured with changes in HR, Wisco et al. (2016) found that, although self-reported BSE was related to better outcome, BSE was not related to more change in PTSD with written exposure therapy. In a study that examined trauma-potentiated startle across PTSD treatment, responders showed an increase in trauma-potentiated startle from baseline to midtreatment followed by a decrease from midtreatment to post-treatment, whereas nonresponders showed a flat response across treatment (Robison-Andrew et al., 2014). In addition, there were no differences between responders and nonresponders in WSE (Robison-Andrew et al., 2014).

CONCLUSION

In summary, emotional activation and WSE have not been well supported in the literature as reliably related to PTSD treatment outcomes following exposure therapy. Of the three proposed indicators of emotional processing, BSE has been the most consistently supported. However, even for BSE the evidence is somewhat mixed for anxiety-related disorders overall, although it has been fairly well supported in studies of PTSD, most of which focus on subjective distress. It may be that BSE is less likely to relate to outcomes in analogue studies that use abbreviated exposure protocols. It may also be that although BSE is common among those with good outcomes, it is not always a reliable indicator of emotional processing in anxiety-related disorders other than PTSD. Finally, methodologically, all the PTSD protocols noted restricted the SUDS and psychophysiological recording to the exposure portion of the session. Because processing is most often discussion and not necessarily close emotional engagement with the memory, most patients have a reduction in anxious arousal prior to the end of the session. No one has examined how patterns during this part of the session relate to outcomes. In addition, for PE, the therapist switches to hot spot exposures at about Session 5 or 6. These briefer exposures typically involve more rapid changes in anxious arousal as the patient works through the most difficult pieces of the memory. Accounting for this waxing-and-waning pattern for the hot spots has not been systematically examined either. Of note, both BSE and WSE are mechanisms of extinction learning theories, but they are not specifically part of emotional processing theory mechanisms of PE.

With advancing technology, psychophysiological recording is becoming cheaper, more accurate, and more portable every day. Indeed, many people now integrate this technology in their life on a regular basis through a Fitbit or Apple Watch. Researchers are always looking for ways to use such real-time and rich data to inform better care through more personalized medicine and more responsive provider training and accessible care. eSense is a commercially available, low-cost, easy-to-use skin conductance monitor that is now being used in clinical care in some settings. Hinrichs et al. (2017) demonstrated that skin conductance collected using eSense during a brief trauma description was predictive of PTSD severity (Wangelin & Tuerk, 2015). This tool is now being used in a research study in an emergency room with acute trauma survivors to determine whether skin conductance can predict PTSD a year after trauma exposure. It is also being used clinically with patients in PTSD treatment (B. O. Rothbaum, personal communication, February 24, 2021; Wangelin & Tuerk, 2015). These tools take the difficulties involved in signal processing out so that providers can use them in real time as they are working with patients in session. For instance, we often use eSense with patients during exposure exercises to see if and how their perceived levels of physiological activation map onto skin conductance. This can help patients see more gradations of emotional activation and early signs of extinction in their emotional responding within and between sessions. Another developing new tool is Stress Analysis by Forward Looking Infrared (FLIR) Evaluation (SAFE). This sensor measures sweat pore reactivity in fingertips, which is highly correlated with skin conductance (Familoni et al., 2016). PTSD patients showed larger response in skin conductance and SAFE to the first startle probe compared with trauma controls and the response correlated with severity of PTSD reexperiencing (Familoni et al., 2016). Although such tools will never replace the precision and specificity of professional psychophysiological monitoring, their use may allow for integration of biomarkers identified with precision tools in the lab to be used in everyday clinical practice. Research continues to expand what we know of how PTSD impacts the brain and body and how treatment is reflected in psychophysiology.

7

GENETICS AND GENOMICS

The *diathesis-stress hypothesis* predominates etiological theory of psychiatric diagnoses. This hypothesis proposes that genetic and environmental adversity provide independent and interactional contributions to psychiatric disorders when a summative threshold that combines the two contributors is crossed. Thus, for some disorders or for some individuals, there can be a small or large genetic contribution, such that the environmental stressor can be the opposite (small or large), resulting in disorder. Within posttraumatic stress disorder (PTSD) this process is two-fold because it requires exposure to an event that meets the definition of trauma and then a reaction to that event that is maintained over time to become PTSD. As summarized below, both exposure to trauma and the development of PTSD have been shown to have genetic and environmental contributors. Over the next 15 years, we are expecting to see an explosion in psychiatric genetics that will be based on the recent, ongoing worldwide collaborations and larger studies, which will provide very large sample sizes with appropriate genetic diversity to allow for better predictions and reliable results. Previous studies have often been plagued by low power and lack of replication across labs and, even, samples within a laboratory.

In this chapter, we discuss some of the most promising techniques being used to provide insight into genetic contributors to exposure to trauma,

https://doi.org/10.1037/0000242-007
Retraining the Brain: Applied Neuroscience in Exposure Therapy for PTSD,
by S. A. M. Rauch and C. P. McLean

reactions to trauma, and PTSD. We move on to present the state of literature regarding genetics and trauma and then genetics and PTSD. Finally, we discuss recent findings and potential contributions of psychiatric genetics to treatment response focusing on PE. Readers are referred to other sources for more comprehensive reviews of psychiatric genetics as it applies to PTSD and anxiety disorders (Morrison et al., 2019; Sharma & Ressler, 2019; Smoller, 2016).

METHODS FOR SCIENTIFIC DISCOVERY

Methods for examination of psychiatric genetics fall into several levels of analysis. In a review, Smoller (2019) indicated six levels for examination as briefly reviewed below. First, examination of whether this disorder was found more frequently in families, using family studies and the *recurrence risk ratio*. This ratio compared the rates of disorders within family members to rates within unaffected families or population prevalence. Although a first step toward showing genetics' influence, these ratios included the familial shared environment and genetic contributions and were thought to provide a high estimate of the genetic contribution. A second level of analysis occured in looking at how much genes contribute to the disorder through twin studies that provided *heritability ratios* or the ratio of the genetic variance (that shared between monozygotic twins) to the full phenotypic variance. The higher the ratios, the larger the genetic contribution to the disorder. The third level uncovered which chromosomes were involved through *linkage studies*. These molecular genetic studies worked to localize and identify the genetic influences at the level of DNA variation to map the areas related to specific disorders. They focused on co-inheritance of DNA markers. Such methods have not borne much fruit for psychiatric disorders that are complex and often not influenced by single markers (Smoller, 2016).

This led to the fourth level of analysis using *association studies*. Association studies are a category of study designs that are more informative for psychiatric disorders that have multiple genetic contributors (Smoller, 2016). These studies used a case-control design to determine which variants (called *alleles*) were more common in people with the disorder (cases) as opposed to those without the disorder (controls). Association studies included several different methods of defining case and control as well as how to examine genetic variations. Single nucleotide polymorphism (SNP; most common variation in adenine, cytosine, guanine, and thymine [ACGT] nucleotides in genetic code) and structural variations (e.g., copy number variants [CNVs], insertions/deletions) are all examples of association study designs. Examination of pathogenic variations (changes arising in the parental gametes or fetus not inherited from previous generations) were also possible (Smoller, 2016).

Association studies are either genome-wide studies or candidate gene studies. *Genome-wide studies* (GWAS) look across the entire genome to find if there are genes present at a significantly higher rate in cases versus controls. These studies often use common SNPs to examine alleles that are correlated or inherited together to reduce the number of comparisons required to examine genome-wide variation. However, even with these techniques, the number of comparisons for GWAS examination requires massive sample sizes that have rarely been available in psychiatric genetics. However, the Psychiatric Genetics Consortium PTSD workgroup is truly changing the landscape of genetics exploration of psychiatric disorders by providing a platform and framework to reach the power required to advance genetic discoveries (Duncan et al., 2018). Candidate gene studies focus analysis on specific genes that have shown association with the disorder in animal studies or previous human studies with more recent candidate gene studies taking genes identified in GWAS and working to replicate in other samples.

In a fifth level of analysis, *gene-by-environment studies* examine whether the impact of genetics varied with environmental stressor exposure (Smoller, 2016). To date, these studies used candidate genes and examined the influence of exposures that have been underpowered. Recent methods, including *polygenic risk scores* (PRS) that provide estimates of aggregate risk across genes in one sample that can be applied to future samples, may offer a more robust analysis of the genetic and gene-by-environment risks (Smoller, 2016). However, recent examination in a military sample over time showed that PRS did not provide main effects or interactions with trauma, PTSD, or depressive symptoms over 5 years (Schür et al., 2019), while another study that did not include longitudinal follow-up did support an association between PRS and PTSD (Y. Wang et al., 2019).

Finally, the sixth level of analysis involved taking the identified gene(s) back to molecular, cellular, and clinical studies to determine how the genes led to the disorder (Smoller, 2016). This was a kind of *reverse engineering* to figure out the interplay of all the influences in the individual case and where in the system intervention can occur to break the cycle of disorder. Additional specifics of psychiatric genetics design are beyond the scope of the current chapter but can be found elsewhere (Morrison et al., 2019; Sharma & Ressler, 2019; Smoller, 2016).

Importantly, with the exception of some large studies conducted out of Detroit and the Grady Trauma Project, much of the research examining genetics has been limited to samples with primarily White European ancestry (for a review, see Sheerin et al., 2017), thus biasing and limiting application of the findings.

WHAT DOES THIS MEAN FOR TRAUMA EXPOSURE AND PTSD?

Many methods are currently in use to examine whether trauma exposure and/ or PTSD may be influenced by genetic or epigenetic factors. This section summarizes key findings using several of the most informative genetic methods.

Family and Twin Studies on Trauma Exposure and PTSD

In a review of genetic research on PTSD and anxiety, Smoller (2019) concluded that risk of PTSD had been found to be elevated in offspring of parents with PTSD. Genetic factors can contribute to PTSD through (a) increasing the likelihood of exposure to criterion A trauma, (b) increasing risk for PTSD symptoms/reactions regardless of trauma exposure, (c) increasing risk factors related to PTSD following trauma (e.g., likelihood to respond through alcohol or substance use or avoidance or other behavioral reactions), or (d) multiple effects from a single gene on any one or combination of the above. This multi-determination adds complexity to the prediction of PTSD.

In his review of research, Smoller (2016) concluded that studies that have examined trauma as the target outcome support that exposure to assaultive and violent trauma, including combat trauma, is heritable, but that nonassaultive trauma (including natural disasters, etc.) appears to be less related or possibly not heritable. On the surface, it may be counterintuitive to think that genes impact experience, but these studies strongly support such an association. Of note, how and why these associations exist are not known. Genes may contribute to personality characteristics, such as risk taking, that may make certain people more likely to encounter trauma, or other factors may intervene. Heritability estimates range from 30% to 50% for PTSD and increase for more high-risk trauma exposures (up to 60%; Duncan et al., 2018; Smoller, 2016). These studies also found that individual PTSD symptoms are heritable (True et al., 1993) and that larger or more frequent doses of trauma can lead to PTSD, even among those with low vulnerability (Jang et al., 2007). Using the Vietnam-Era Twin Study Registry, E. J. Wolf et al. (2014) found that the associations between genetic predictors and PTSD was highest among those with the highest reported levels of combat exposure. Of note, further analyses in this registry also found support for consideration of a continuum of vulnerability between PTSD and resilience in heritability, rather than examining these constructs orthogonally. Specifically, the overlap of heritability between PTSD and resilience in this sample was high and suggested that the same contributors were at work (E. J. Wolf et al., 2018). Additional work is needed to confirm whether these constructs are a continuum or separate.

Candidate Gene Studies and Genome-Wide Association Studies (GWAS)

Many candidate genes have been examined with focus on systems identified as being involved in stress response and anxiety, including many related to hypothalamic–pituitary–adrenal (HPA) axis function, inflammation, and monaniergic and opiodergic neurotransmission, with few surviving replication (Smoller, 2016). For instance, a meta-analysis of studies examining the serotonin transporter gene polymorphism *5HTTLPR*, which is common in European ancestry cohorts, found no evidence of an association outside of high trauma exposure samples (Gressier et al., 2013). While many other genes have been implicated in single studies or smaller samples, larger ongoing studies and replications of these nominal associations are underway to establish these associations. As a result, they will not be described here, but readers are encouraged to explore more focused reviews on the topic (Morrison et al., 2019; Sharma & Ressler, 2019; Smoller, 2016).

Although extensive review of all genetic studies to date is beyond the scope of this chapter, recent reviews conclude that a few genes stand out on the basis of candidate gene studies: C-reactive protein (*CRP*), a variant in the opioid receptor-like 1 gene (OPRL1), pituitary adenylate cyclase-activating polypeptide (PACAP), *FK506* binding protein 5 gene (*FKBP5*), and vesicular monoamine transporter 2 (VMAT2; Sheerin et al., 2017; Smoller, 2016). These genes are highlighted on the basis of replications across different samples combined with follow-on molecular, cellular, and clinical studies that support the biological processes involved in conferring risk. For instance, variants of the *CRP* gene were found to be associated with higher PTSD among high trauma exposed African Americans in the Grady Trauma Project study (Michopoulos et al., 2015). These risk SNPs were determined to be associated with higher serum *CRP* levels, which were in turn related to more severe PTSD symptoms and fear potentiated startle (Michopoulos et al., 2015). Although these candidate genes stand out, many of them are predictors only among subpopulations (e.g., highly traumatized African Americans). Additional work is needed to extend these findings to other relevant groups.

The Psychiatric Genetics Consortium PTSD workgroup recently published the largest GWAS study of PTSD to date (Duncan et al., 2018). They found significant heritability of PTSD for European American women (29%), but not for men, and significant overlap in this heritability with schizophrenia, followed by bipolar disorder and major depressive disorder (Duncan et al., 2018). This overlap with other disorders is important as the field determines what are the factors related to general mental health difficulty versus specific manifestations, such as PTSD versus panic disorder. It is highly likely that the genetic underpinning of many mental health issues is shared with expression determined by environmental factors or even chance. Of note, no SNPs reached significance in this transethnic analysis. Similarly, K. Zhang et al. (2017) compiled a PTSD gene genetic database of 105 PTSD studies and concluded that PTSD shares the most candidate genes with schizophrenia (45 genes).

Gene-Environment Interaction

In a review of gene-by-environment studies, DiGangi et al. (2013) concluded that little has been determined to be conclusive, because most of these studies have been underpowered and restricted to small groups of polymorphisms, without attention to timing, chronicity, and differential effect sizes. Two gene-by-environment interactions that have been replicated are the PACAP receptor (Almli et al., 2013; Ressler et al., 2011; Uddin et al., 2013) and the promoter region of a polymorphism in the B2 adrenergic gene (Liberzon et al., 2014). In addition, a compelling program of research has provided support for a mechanism of action for the association between childhood adversity and *FKBP5* polymorphism. This program of research includes examination of the molecular basis for *FKBP5* genotype interacting with childhood trauma to induce epigenetically mediated hippocampal glucocorticoid resistance; it supports the role of sensitive periods (trauma occurring outside of that period is not associated with the same cascade of events) and the importance of different types of adversity in their impact (chronic adversity that can occur through neglect, poor nutrition, etc. vs. acute incidents of trauma; Klengel et al., 2013; Zannas & Binder, 2014).

WHAT DOES THIS MEAN FOR PE?

Genetics in PTSD have not yet provided specific treatment direction. Indeed, little research has examined genetic factors as they relate to treatment response in PTSD and even less specifically as they are relevant to PE. Studies are currently ongoing to explore whether genetic factors can predict treatment response (e.g., S. A. M. Rauch et al., 2018). Previous chapters that have examined psychophysiological and other neurobiological processes as they relate to PTSD likely all have genetic contributors. As we discover more clearly how these processes work, we can also discover genetic contributors. Conversely, as we discover genetic contributors, additional research looking at the mechanisms of how those genes confer risk can inform our knowledge of PTSD and its treatment. The advent of new tools—such as transcriptomics and proteomics that involve looking at how gene expression differs across conditions, systems, and over time—can inform this progress.

PART **III** APPLIED
NEUROSCIENCE:
PROLONGED
EXPOSURE
FOR PTSD

8 PSYCHOEDUCATION AND NEUROSCIENCE

The three key components of prolonged exposure (PE) are *psychoeducation*, *in vivo exposure*, and *imaginal exposure with processing* as presented in the second edition of the therapist manual (Foa, Hembree, et al., 2019). In Part III, then, we take a closer look at these components in relation to applied neuroscience.

We begin, in this chapter, with the foundation of PE in psychoeducation. This critical component of PE provides the grounding on which the rest of the work can grow. Although most of the psychoeducation is provided in Sessions 1 through 3, additional psychoeducation can occur as needed throughout treatment. This can include (a) repetition of previous content, (b) reflection of specific experiences that the patient has that are consistent with the psychoeducation, or (c) specific additional information to help discuss how the treatment is working for this specific patient. If the grounding is firm and stable, the patient may still feel anxious to do the work of PE but will feel able to take the chance on the intervention. If the grounding is not firm and stable, the patient may feel less able to take the chance to approach, instead of avoiding, the trauma memory and reminders, as is required in PE. Directly connecting this to previously presented neuroscience, the more a patient feels a sense of control over what they are doing in PE sessions and for homework, the less the likelihood of overactivation of the stress response system. As presented

https://doi.org/10.1037/0000242-008
Retraining the Brain: Applied Neuroscience in Exposure Therapy for PTSD,
by S. A. M. Rauch and C. P. McLean

in Chapter 3, perceived control is a robust predictor of the release of cortisol and hypothalamic–pituitary–adrenal (HPA) axis response (Bollini et al., 2004) and lower coritsol response to full trauma memories is related to better PE outcomes (Norrholm et al., 2016). The exposures will be difficult for patients with posttraumatic stress disorder (PTSD), but the more they understand treatment and how we think it works, the more they will be willing to try and the more they will stay with difficult exposures to get the benefits of new learning.

ESTABLISHING THE FOUNDATION

Although there are many key points of psychoeducation presented in the first few sessions of PE, the core points of PE psychoeducation are: (a) PTSD is developed and maintained because of avoidance and unhelpful trauma-related thoughts about the self and the world; (b) repeatedly approaching and revisiting that trauma memory will help organize and provide the opportunity for new perspectives on what happened during and after the trauma; (c) repeatedly revisiting the trauma memory will differentiate "remembering" the trauma from the possibility of actually experiencing the trauma again; (d) repeated imaginal exposure that includes staying with the memory for an adequate amount of time (about 40 minutes) allows for reduction of the intensity of negative emotions connected with the memory; (e) the patient experiences this reduction of intensity when they approach the trauma memory and they do not lose control, "go crazy," or "fall apart"; and (f) repeatedly recounting the trauma memory increases patients' sense of self-control and personal competence.

Psychoeducation provides information on how PE works but, just as important, provides a context of trust and hope that fuels therapeutic change. When providing the information, it is not necessary or even desirable that the patient understand all the findings of neuroscience as it relates to treatment. Turning a therapy session into a neuroscience course is unlikely to result in better outcomes and takes time and effort away from the key therapy components. However, giving the patient a foundation with some level of understanding for why you will be asking them to do things that are difficult is important. As such, sticking with the tested PE psychoeducation model is likely the best way to start PE. What we know from neuroscience can be brought to bear in the moments of difficulty or impasse, when the patient may be stuck or motivation is waning because of high anticipatory anxiety or challenging exposures, specifically to give the patient a greater sense of control as noted above. As a provider, if you understand how neuroscience maps onto emotional processing theory, inhibitory learning, and extinction learning, you may better reflect those concepts in discussion or better answer patient questions as they arise. Starting with explanation of the neurocircuitry model of PTSD as applied to PE builds in delay before the experience of exposure, and such delay is counterproductive. Such attempts require time in an already packed first or second PE session. However, when the patient encounters a tough in vivo or imaginal exposure session, a savvy therapist can then add specific description based on what we know about neuroscience and PE. Being able to smoothly bring up a relevant point can be powerful. For instance, consider a patient who completed their first imaginal exposure session with good engagement and activation of the memory who now does not want to do it again. A short discussion of how repeated activation of the memory is needed in order to strengthen the new extinction learning connections to the point that the brain more strongly connects the memory with safety over threat may encourage the patient to continue with imaginal exposure.

One key point in psychoeducation is that therapists suggest the direction and provide support but allow the patients to set the course. This is important in working with patients with PTSD, where a sense of competence and control is important. Ensuring that patients feel they are driving the course of therapy helps enhance their feelings of accomplishment as they do the exposures that are part of treatment and helps them feel safe because they know they can always change course if they feel that is needed. As such, when patients indicate that a therapist is "making" them do an exposure or stay in an exposure, it is important for the provider to address this gently and remind them that they can stop at any time, while also reminding them of the goal of the exposure.

As you recall from previous chapters, context matters in learning. Providing a therapeutic context that allows for new learning is critical to retention in therapy and critical for new learning to occur robustly. This does not suggest a therapeutic context without affect but, rather, a context where affect can be expressed and experienced to allow for reduction of intensity and learning that the patient can handle the negative affect. This therapeutic context begins with building rapport in psychoeducation. In addition, as described in Chapter 4 on imaging, learning contextualization involves the hippocampus, HPA axis (dorsal anterior cingulate), and other brain structures. Building rapport means building trust. Trust is built through active listening and reflection of the patient's experience within and across sessions. For instance, if, during the initial assessment, the patient mentioned that he is only attending sessions because he wants to attend his daughter's softball games, then making sure this is included as one of the exposures listed on the in vivo exposure hierarchy (as a target for treatment) can aid in the patient feeling motivated for treatment and validated. When patients know that you are listening to their priorities, they will more likely believe that you are listening to their more difficult and complex thoughts and feelings. The PE therapist must ensure that patients feel heard and build on the patient's experience and what matters to them.

Rapport can also grow through statements of sincere affirmation for patients' courage in considering approaching, rather than avoiding, their trauma memory and reminders and through therapist statements that align with patients in this mission. For instance, the therapist might state, "Thank you for coming to your session today. I can hear that you were feeling anxious about our session, but you came anyway. This is a step toward taking your life back from PTSD." Such statements put the therapist and patient on the same side of the fight against PTSD, and this provides a new context of safety that can be incorporated into the imaginal exposure memory. Such connections can facilitate PE through increasing social support and possibly facilitating the associated neurochemical processes related to social support that also facilitate learning (Donadon et al., 2018; Price et al., 2013), as well as through increasing a sense of perceived control (Bollini et al., 2004).

In addition to building rapport, instilling hope is another function of psychoeducation. Instilling hope through providing an expectation of recovery and a path to make recovery a reality is important in the early sessions of PE. Patients will be better able to stick with the negative affect of the trauma memory and reminders if they know there is something better coming. The more specific that benefit can be, the more the therapist can connect to it when tough sessions occur. With the patient who said he was only here so that he could attend his daughter's softball games, for instance, reminding him during tough imaginal exposure sessions that this goal or motivation is a path to how he can reduce the interference and take his life back from PTSD can help maintain motivation. Letting a patient know about the experience of previous patients who were symptomatic, completed PE, and can now do the things they want to in life can also be helpful. For patients who may be on the fence, referring them to specific PE success videos online (e.g., www.aboutface.org or www.maketheconnection.org) can go a long way to letting them know that this form of therapy can work. Although several effective treatments are available, we also know that there is a lot of room for improvement in retention and magnitude of change. However, trauma-focused therapy remains the best first-line treatment, with estimates of about 40% remission for those who complete a course and with many others receiving significant benefit. At the very least, such efforts increase willingness to engage in PE and to continue in PE long enough to receive an effective "dose." Additional research using the latest tools of neuroscience is needed to more effectively operationalize what "dose" is required.

When therapists show their confidence in the treatment, patients can borrow that confidence until they begin to experience it themselves. From a neuroscience perspective, your reactions as the therapist and your presence in the room as patients approach the memory in imaginal exposure are both providing content for the new extinction memory that is being created and strengthening with repetition. This means that your tone of voice, your systematic and confident process to ask for subjective units of distress (SUDS) and provide an encouraging statement every 5 minutes, and so forth can all provide pieces of a new extinction memory that demonstrates mastery of the trauma memory, including its emotional content. When connecting this to the previously presented findings, therapists can consider how their reactions may pull the patient away from their trauma memory and into the present. For instance, many patients have never verbally recalled their trauma memories in the presence of another person. Indeed, this shared experience has been suggested as a possible therapeutic element of PE (S. A. M. Rauch et al., 2019). If the therapist's reaction projects safety and acceptance of the experience, the patient can remain connected with the memory and this safety learning becomes part of the new trauma memory (as discussed in the previous chapters). If, however, the therapist's reaction projects judgment (e.g., gasping, appearing shocked), then that safety context is not present, and patients may even disengage the memory to try and reduce perceived therapist negative reactions.

LEARNING UNDER STRESS

In PTSD treatment that includes PE, we ask patients to learn under the worst conditions for learning to occur—that is, while experiencing high anxiety (Vogel & Schwabe, 2016). As such, patient repetition should be expected and built into everything the PE therapist does to repeatedly try until the patient overlearns the target rather than just gets "good enough." This means continuing to repeat treatment if there is any doubt of whether the patient has fully "processed" the memory. In the context of PE, "processing" refers to approaching the memory in such a way that emotional intensity is reduced, that meaning is altered in a therapeutic direction, and that the patient feels better able to handle the memory and related emotions in the present and, possibly, even feel they have handled it better in the past than they originally thought. Although learning is more difficult and often requires more repetition with high anxiety, it may also make spontaneous recovery of the trauma memory (where intrusive symptoms of the memory return after an initial reduction) less likely (Singewald & Holmes, 2019). Thus, when learned, such associations are retained better over time.

Therapists can be efficient and effective by providing useful information at a digestible level, so that patients get a gist of how PE works and why they are being asked to approach trauma-related stimuli instead of avoiding them. Then they can incorporate more specific or advanced information when needed, as the patient proceeds through PE. Think of it as a scaffold provided by standard PE psychoeducation. For some patients, this may be all they need to take off and make it to the top. For other patients, additional information may be needed to build out the scaffold to allow them to reach the top. Such information may include discussions about their personal patterns of SUDS in their imaginal exposure sessions and what that pattern may indicate. For instance, the therapist might explicitly reflect back to patients that they are showing a reduction in SUDS. For other patients, the therapist might explicitly reflect back that, although patients did not show reduction in SUDS, they stayed with the exposure despite high SUDS for a longer duration (i.e., they tolerated the distress). Both patterns can indicate helpful learning, but a therapist may choose to talk about them differently. When intensity is reduced, this is the "classic" habituation pattern, and when the patient's tolerance is increased in staying with the imaginal for more time despite high intensity, this may indicate distress tolerance or inhibitory learning. Both of these effects may be relevant to highlight or discuss with the patient, with the key explicit learning point being that the patient is approaching, instead of avoiding, the trauma memory and reminders, an achievement that will allow them to get back to doing the things in life that they want to do again.

AVOIDING RELAPSE

Relapse prevention begins before we even start therapy with a patient. When providers set expectations for patients about the focus of treatment, what they will be working on, what they will not be working on, and what outcome can be expected, they set the groundwork for relapse prevention. All these pieces can set a context that primes the patient for therapeutic change. Ensuring that patients have a clear understanding of how to apply the principles of exposure on their own for generalization and maintenance of gains is one way to reduce the risk of relapse. This starts not only with the basic understanding of the rationale for imaginal and in vivo exposure but may also include a discussion with the patient about that individual's personal learning style and pattern of habituation/extinction while they have engaged in care. Neuroscience tells us that continued repetition of new learning can make the learning more robust to spontaneous recovery. In clinical terms, this means that repeating exposures until they are truly boring (and maybe even a little more thereafter) can help prevent future situations in which the old trauma memory might reemerge—such as under life stress or experiences that are similar to the trauma.

Neuroscience can play a role in PE psychoeducation. Although this does not change the standard protocol for PE and psychoeducation from the manual, it can serve as a discussion point or additional points of support to enhance the patient's experience in PE and can be used to increase retention and reduce relapse. When patients know that what they are feeling across treatment is "normal," they are often more motivated to continue to progress through treatment. Additional neuroscience research is currently underway (e.g., breaking down how PE works) and can further inform PE practice.

9 IN VIVO EXPOSURE AND NEUROSCIENCE

In vivo exposure in prolonged exposure (PE) is a core component and a primary part of recovery. Through in vivo exposures, patients begin to take their lives back from posttraumatic stress disorder (PTSD), as they approach rather than avoid the people, places, and situations that are associated with their trauma. Thinking back to Chapters 1 and 2 of this book and with reference to the PE manual (Foa, Hembree, et al., 2019), the hierarchy for in vivo exposure may include items that are associated with the trauma and provoke negative affective responses, as well as items that may be associated with behavioral activation whose goal is to reconnect with the world and community. In this chapter, we focus on how to make neuroscience-informed decisions in practice when using in vivo exposure to optimize patient outcomes that are based on what we know about how PE works in the brain and the body.

NEUROSCIENCE APPLIED TO HIERARCHY PLANNING

Choosing which items to include on a hierarchy is critical to the success and impact of PE. A therapist who is not effective in building a powerful hierarchy with a patient will be less effective in reducing PTSD. As noted above, in vivo

https://doi.org/10.1037/0000242-009
Retraining the Brain: Applied Neuroscience in Exposure Therapy for PTSD,
by S. A. M. Rauch and C. P. McLean

exposure is the tool that most specifically gets patients back doing the things that they want to do in life. The most effective PE therapists begin with the end goal in mind, which means that they are including items on the hierarchy with consideration of the goal for each planned individual exposure exercise. For each hierarchy item, therapists should consider two questions: What is the core fear that the item is addressing? What specific learning does the patient need to get from this in vivo item? To illustrate, driving in heavy traffic is an item on many combat PTSD hierarchies. However, an effective therapist who is using neuroscience to inform PE practice is considering the specifics of this in vivo scenario in detail. If the core fear is that the patient would be trapped and unable to escape, the specific variations on this item would be different than if the core fear is that potholes cannot be seen in traffic and represent an urgent threat. Variations for the first core fear would include ensuring that the patient has varying levels of being surrounded by traffic (feeling more or less trapped). The second situation would involve varying the likelihood of encountering potholes. The most effective hierarchies are made up of items (a) where the patients can see and feel the impact on their daily functioning and quality of life, (b) that increase social connection and reduce isolation, (c) that include variations to allow for specific experiences of generalization, and (d) that allow systematic repetition of the core fear/ negative affect outcome.

Unpacking each of these items and connecting to the core neuroscience findings reviewed in Part I of this book, we begin with the concept of preferentially including those items where patients can see and feel the impact on their daily function and quality of life. The obvious reason for this is that people come to treatment to address a problem (e.g., I cannot attend my child's sporting events; I cannot enjoy sexual relations with my partner). When providers can make changes that address the presenting problem, patients experience increased motivation, hope for additional positive changes, and so forth. These changes are reflected in lower symptoms, more confidence, and more positive thoughts about themselves and the world (e.g., Foa & Rauch, 2004; Kumpula et al., 2017; McLean, Yeh, et al., 2015; McLean et al., 2019; Zalta et al., 2014), as well as in changes in body responses, such as heart racing or sweating (e.g., Maples-Keller, Rauch, et al., 2019; S. A. M. Rauch, King, et al., 2015). Indeed, we would expect that as patients experience mastery in situations that they previously avoided because of their association with trauma, these bodily changes and self-perceptions create a positive change feedback loop that can increase outcomes and motivation to continue to work hard in treatment. As patients do the things they want to do, they are happier, healthier, and farther along in recovery.

Why does neuroscience suggest that we include items that enhance social connection and reduce social isolation? Research supports the beneficial impact of positive social connection on mood possibly through oxytocin (Donadon et al., 2018). Whereas results of augmentation studies of PE with oxytocin have been mixed with a current trial ongoing, the psychotherapy literature suggests that social support is one of the most reliable predictors of positive treatment response (Dour et al., 2014; Price et al., 2013). In addition, connection to family, community, and loved ones provides buffering from relapse, as well as motivation for new life goals and meaning (S. A. M. Rauch, Yasinski, et al., 2020). Thus, therapists can encourage specific opportunities for prosocial connections during PE that would likely increase the release of oxytocin through incorporation of items in the in vivo hierarchy that involve social interactions with family, friends, and community. For instance, PE therapists may encourage a patient who experienced combat trauma to approach military memorabilia and join a veteran organization where such materials are displayed. This would address both extinction to the activation associated with military memorabilia and allow for social and community connection.

Generalization of PE learning is critical to improving functioning. Indeed, in life, generalization is the process in which a patient takes the specific exposure experience and applies it in new settings in different ways. This may involve a conscious process in which a patient may explicitly verbalize or think about the generalization. For instance, a patient who avoided grocery shopping may complete in vivo exposures that involve going to a specific grocery store. After treatment, that patient may say that they are only safe in that store, that chain of stores, or all grocery stores. These different statements, then, would reflect different types of generalization and relate to magnitude of symptoms reduction. The more widely patients apply the new learning, the more patients are able to do the things they want to do in life and make choices out of situational needs instead of trauma-related anxiety. In neuroscience as applied to PE, generalization is the specific expansion of extinction learning to relevant, although not identical, stimuli. As discussed in Part I, generalization gradients can be used to operationalize how widely a specific learned association is applied. When considering the extinction learning that is part of PE, therapists doing in vivo exposure are typically trying to promote maximal generalization, so that previously feared people, places, and situations are no longer considered dangerous and are now associated with safety. As such, it is important for the therapist to consider strategies to increase generalization that will provide the most benefit to the patient. This means systematically considering what variations of a specific in vivo item will be beneficial for this individual, with an eye toward making modifications to the plan based on patient response. Variations to ensure generalization should begin with an understanding of the core fear that drives the avoidance and then include different versions of situations that hit that core fear. These variations may include lower or higher levels of the core fear stimulus (e.g., more or less frequent potholes), time of day, being with people or on one's own, and so on.

Finally, neuroscience of extinction learning supports that in vivo hierarchy items may be most effective when they allow for systematic repetition of the core fear/negative affect outcome. This repetition increases the likelihood of extinction and inhibitory learning processes. Extinction learning models support that increased repetition is related to lower spontaneous recovery (Singewald & Holmes, 2019) and would expect this to extend to exposure therapy.

ACTIVATION DURING IN VIVO EXPOSURE PRACTICE

Ensuring that in vivo exposures are maximally effective begins with working to identify and make specific the target of each in vivo. What is the core fear or negative consequence that drives the specific avoidance? How can the patient approach that feared consequence, stay with the emotional responses it provokes for a reasonable period, and repeat it many times? Sometimes the answers to these questions are not entirely clear before the first attempt at an in vivo. In such cases, it can be good for the therapist to take the stance of a scientist or detective, whereby they approach the situation and collect the needed information to refine the exposure to be even more effective subsequently. For instance, a patient who has not been to a movie in a theater for a while may not remember whether the aisle or the center seats are related to more anxiety/fear, but if they can test it out they can know for certain. An important piece of in vivo exposure is discussion of the experience with the therapist. (In-depth discussion of processing and ways to facilitate processing are presented in Chapter 11.) For our current discussion, processing incudes discussing how the in vivo exposure went, whether it was harder or easier and why, what the patient learned from the exposure, and what they still need to learn. On the basis of how processing went, the exposure can be fine-tuned to target the specific feared consequence. For instance, if it becomes clear that a critical element was not present and the resulting in vivo was too easy, then that element can be added. An example of this may be a rape survivor who is doing exposure to crowded stores and reports a subjective units of distress (SUDS) rating of 50 and then discovers, during discussion, that she went with her partner, which made it easier. The next iteration of the in vivo item would specifically have her going shopping on her own and discussing the difference.

Neuroscience also provides important direction for therapists that between-session reductions in SUDS and psychophysiological arousal, but not within-session reductions, are most closely related to better outcomes (G.-J. Hendriks et al., 2015; S. A. M. Rauch et al., 2004; S. A. M. Rauch, King, et al., 2015). Even for between-session reduction, there is also evidence that the reduction in distress may be related to, but not necessarily required for, therapeutic benefit in PE—which is suggestive of inhibitory learning and affect tolerance (Bluett et al., 2014). In this way, when a patient is showing within-session changes, it can be a "bonus" support for progress; all the same, the therapist should focus discussion more on whether reductions in distress and arousal are happening across repetitions in time. If such patterns are not apparent, the therapist can look for common impediments to exposure, such as safety behaviors, not staying in the session long enough for the consequence to be felt, not repeating the exposure often enough to see benefit, or not being consistent enough in the exposure for it to feel like repetition. Sometimes it can be helpful to have many repetitions together, often called *massed exposure*, or to space the repetitions out. Massed presentations tend to be best for those exposures that the patient is having a tough time accomplishing until they begin to see some benefit. *Spaced exposures* tend to be good for continued practice and maintenance of gains over time. Finally, therapists should be watching for chances to vary exposures in order to work on generalization (as previously discussed).

Although *underengagement* (or low activation) is more common, some patients may emotionally connect with the memory so closely that they lose connection with the here-and-now, or they are not able to incorporate corrective information in the memory. This is called *overengagement*. In addition to those patients who overengage, some are afraid of losing control, which prevents them from connecting with the trauma memory. Preparatory interventions developed to get patients "ready" for PE have shown some evidence of efficacy, but research designs to date have not compared standard PE to these interventions (Beidel et al., 2011; Cloitre et al., 2010). In addition, any observed benefits of preparatory treatment must be weighed against possible negative effects of extending the course of treatment (increased dropout) and delaying exposure.

DISCRIMINATING SAFETY FROM THREAT

In previous chapters, we discussed the importance of context in extinction learning that is a critical element of PE. As noted in Chapters 1 and 2, people with PTSD show an overgeneralization of fear learning (Morey et al., 2015) and more context-dependence in extinction learning (Liberzon & Abelson, 2016). As such, specifically and explicitly discussing safety and the limits of safety, as in vivo exposures are planned and completed, can help to overcome this tendency and increase the potency of a given in vivo exposure. To demonstrate, this can be as simple as talking with the trauma survivor about specific items being placed on the hierarchy and discussing whether these avoided situations would be avoided by their neighbors or peers. Such types of questions can help patients step out of their perspective for a moment to consider another way of viewing the risks in the world. Once this discussion occurs, then, together, patient and therapist can come to consensus on the relative risk of the situation. Of note for any exposure therapist, the goal is not to declare safety or risk, because we have to recognize not only that bad things can happen anywhere and at any time, but that each person needs to decide what level of risk they are willing to take on in order to have a life that is fulfilling. The level of risk for those with PTSD has been contaminated by their experience of trauma, and the job of therapists is to help them reconsider relative risk to decide a new normal that can work for them.

As we learn more about how PTSD develops and how PE works to treat PTSD in the brain and body, applying the cutting-edge research in clinical practice helps us increase magnitude or efficiency of response to a given session or whole treatment course. In doing so we may even be able to increase retention and response and expand the number of people impacted with PTSD who can achieve remission and reclaim their loves following trauma. In vivo exposure is the tool in PE that most specifically helps people suffering with PTSD to approach those activities that they used to do but that they now avoid due to trauma. Each step is a step toward function and freedom from the impact of PTSD.

10 IMAGINAL EXPOSURE AND NEUROSCIENCE

The core of prolonged exposure (PE) is imaginal (trauma memory) exposure, and neuroscience research and theory is highly relevant to the best practice of imaginal exposure in session. We begin here with key issues in the standard practice of imaginal exposure in PE. Then, we provide additional expansion on common clinical issues of over- and underengagement. In addition, we discuss how neuroscience and theory can be used to make decisions about how to apply imaginal exposure to increase speed and magnitude of response to each imaginal exposure session and, thus, maximize patient outcome and maintenance over time.

ACTIVATION

As discussed in previous chapters, activation of the trauma memory is necessary for effective PE (S. A. M. Rauch & Foa, 2006). In Chapter 6, we reviewed the literature relevant to whether the peak of activation is related to outcome, concluding that evidence is equivocal but generally supports that better engagement with the trauma memory, including the emotional content in early sessions of imaginal exposure, produces better outcomes. In addition, patients

https://doi.org/10.1037/0000242-010
Retraining the Brain: Applied Neuroscience in Exposure Therapy for PTSD,
by S. A. M. Rauch and C. P. McLean

who do not engage with the emotional content of their trauma memories during imaginal exposure, as measured with psychophysiological and neuroendocrine activation, tend to show less reduction in posttraumatic stress disorder (PTSD) symptoms (Foa et al., 1995; Pitman et al., 1996; S. A. M. Rauch, King, et al., 2015; Wangelin & Tuerk, 2015). Studies using subjective reports of distress have been more equivocal, with some supporting higher activation being related to better outcome (Jaycox et al., 1998) while others do not (Bluett et al., 2004; van Minnen & Hagenaars, 2002). Because the weight of the evidence falls toward activation of emotional content during early imaginal exposures as good, neuroscience can provide insights into how to "jump start" imaginal exposure to increase efficiency of exposures for all patients or to apply specific strategies for patients who may not activate as easily in the first session.

The first strategy of standard PE is to probe for emotional content during imaginal exposure. Probes should be (a) brief, (b) in the present tense, (c) emotion or specific-detail focused, and (d) about the present moment that the patient is describing. Asking double-barreled questions or inquiring about complex thoughts pulls the patient away from being present with the memory and reduces activation. Asking probes such as "What are you thinking?," "What emotion are you feeling?," or "What does his face look like?," however, can help avoidant patients remember to include important content.

A second well-supported strategy to increase activation and boost the learning that occurs in imaginal exposure is to start with a probe. Standard PE would not suggest doing this routinely. Most patients will not require such probes to connect with the memory. Allowing the patient to lead the first imaginal exposure has general benefit in their increase in sense of competence to manage the memory. However, if a patient is underengaged (low activation of the memory where it is not present during imaginal exposure) or is not progressing in imaginal exposure over time, exposure to specific stimulus probes from the target trauma memory prior to or during imaginal exposure can be helpful. *Virtual reality exposure* (VRE) *therapy* is based on this idea of providing the visual, auditory, and olfactory cues of the trauma context, so that the patient is already immersed at the start of the imaginal exposure (Loucks et al., 2019). Without using VRE, there are still many options for probes. Neuroscience suggests that, on the basis of connections between olfaction and emotion processing in the brain, olfactory probes may be especially robust (Soudry et al., 2011), but specific studies examining augmentation with olfactory cues in PE have not yet been conducted. Despite this, many providers suggest that underengaged patients bring smells associated with the trauma into the room. For patients with war-related PTSD, some common olfactory cues include the smell of blood, which can be cued by having patients hold and smell pennies in their hand, body odor and smells that approximate burnt flesh, and other critical trauma elements. Smelling these cues prior to or during imaginal exposure often moves patients to connect with the memory more fully. In addition, for patients who are not having trouble with underengagement, such cues can be good targets for in vivo exposure if avoiding them affects patient function.

Another strategy to increase activation for imaginal exposure that is informed by neuroscience is to provide a behavioral or pharmacological intervention to increase physiological indicators of emotional activation during imaginal exposure. As established in the classic study of Schachter and Singer (1962) and articulated in their *two-factor theory of emotion*, when emotional activation occurs, our brains attempt to explain and label the activation. For example, the same heart rate increase could be attributed to love or fear, depending on contextual information. Thus, if patients who are having a hard time feeling the emotions connected to their trauma memory precede imaginal exposure with exercise or with a medication such as yohimbine (which increases heart rate), they may attribute the resulting arousal to be connected to the imaginal exposure and begin to feel the trauma-related emotions more fully, leading to improved outcomes. As reviewed in the previous chapters, preliminary data suggest that this may be the case (e.g., Powers et al., 2015; Tuerk et al., 2018). In addition, on the basis of research supporting that exercise enhances extinction learning in rats via brain-derived neurotrophic factor (BDNF), Powers et al. (2015) showed that BDNF levels were increased and PTSD reductions enhanced in PTSD patients who received PE plus exercise as compared with those who got PE alone. Thus, exercise may increase the availability of endogenous neurochemicals that can enhance the impact of each imaginal exposure session.

EXTINCTION AND INHIBITORY LEARNING IN IMAGINAL EXPOSURE

As noted in Chapter 6 on psychophysiology, there is evidence to support that both classical extinction learning and inhibitory learning occur in imaginal exposure in PE. We will not review that literature again here but will highlight key findings as they apply to the practice of imaginal exposure in PE. Inhibitory learning is a model of extinction learning developed most notably by Craske et al. (2014) that advances our understanding of how extinction includes more than just a simple reduction in the association between the conditioned stimulus and the unconditioned stimulus.

Research on extinction learning and retention models support that extinction creates a new memory that competes with the old fear memory when cues in the environment are present. Whether the extinction memory or fear memory "wins" (i.e., is recalled in any given context) is dependent on relative activation strength or whether the extinction memory has been learned robustly enough to prevent the fear expression. An extinction memory is learned robustly when the competing safety cues associated with it are numerous and certain enough for the patient to have a sense of relative safety or that there is a manageable amount of risk (Craske et al., 2014; Paredes & Morilak, 2019). For imaginal exposure this means that increased repetition can increase effectiveness, as well as ensure that as many trauma cues are present in the imaginal as possible. Any cues that are connected with the trauma should be included in the imaginal exposure so that the extinction memory includes those cues. Further, the imaginal exposures would ideally continue until the emotional activation is reduced or until the patient feels able to handle the negative affect that is produced when the trauma memory is activated. Applying this specifically to hot spot exposures, therapists should work to ensure that patients truly express all of the affect associated with the hot spots, because this can enhance the sense of ability to handle the affect associated with the trauma memory and provides ample opportunity for repetition of the most relevant trauma cues.

In addition to providing a new extinction memory with a more therapeutic context, the learning that occurs during imaginal exposure needs to generalize outside of the session. In PE, listening to the imaginal exposure outside of the session can provide both increased repetition and generalization so that the patient can approach and experience the trauma memory and emotions *within* the session with a therapist present and *outside* the session when the patient is alone. Often overlooked, this is an important part of what patients learn in PE. Specifically, emotions are not dangerous. Memories are not dangerous. In addition to varying at home and in the office, new protocols such as PE for primary care (Cigrang et al., 2017) also provide variation in how the memory is approached (written and verbal), because both protocols have patients write their trauma and then read it with the therapist. This may provide additional generalization. Therapists may further encourage generalization by recommending incorporating variation in at-home exposures by practicing at different times of day, when arousal may vary, or other contextual variables.

Imaging research shows that patients with PTSD show a globally reduced ability to use contextual information to modulate fear expression (Garfinkel et al., 2014). Specifically, PTSD patients do not notice or attend to stimuli in situations that may signal safety as opposed to danger. For example, a patient with PTSD sees all trips to the crowded grocery store as equally dangerous, but someone without PTSD would notice that the crowded store may be safer at certain times of day or when the store is in a lower crime area. Thus, during imaginal exposure the therapist can help facilitate progress through inclusion of key contextual details in the repetition—such as those variables that may have led to the trauma happening or to the patient surviving the trauma, as well as those details that increased the traumatic impact. For a rape survivor, this may be the size and method of attack of the rapist. For the combat trauma survivor, this may be the chaos of an ambush or the presence of other troops at the time of the improvised explosive device (IED) detonation. Hearing these details in the imaginal exposure may be important elements to include in the extinction memory that is created and competes with the trauma memory. In addition, these contextual details can be important for the processing that follows imaginal exposure (see Chapter 11).

On the basis of the importance of extinction in PE, several studies have been conducted, with mixed results, using medications that are thought to enhance learning (de Kleine et al., 2012; Difede et al., 2014; Rothbaum et al., 2014). Recent reviews have suggested that more precise studies are needed that ensure therapeutic dosing with appropriate timing before or after sessions and even applied only after sessions where significant learning has been accomplished (J. F. Baker et al., 2017).

Of note, recent studies have begun to identify predictors of treatment response trajectories for PE that may help to identify specific patients who may benefit from augmentation or enhancements to PE protocol. For instance, some such studies support that patients who show less than a 10-point reduction in PTSD symptoms (on the basis of the PTSD checklist) by Session 8 of PE may benefit from augmentation or alternate treatment plans (Blow et al., 2019; Ready et al., 2018; Sripada et al., 2020). In addition, several promising biomarkers of a slower treatment trajectory have been identified at baseline (e.g., Norrholm et al., 2016; S. A. M. Rauch, King, et al., 2015; S. A. M. Rauch et al., 2020a, 2020b).

Applied neuroscience can give a PE therapist additional tools to use in the effective implementation of imaginal exposure. As noted above, emphasizing repetition, connection with affect, reductions in emotion activation over time as well as increased tolerance to handle affect activation are all key points of emphasis in the effective application of PE. Using our evolving understanding of the underlying learning processes involved in effective treatment to increase efficiency and effectiveness of each exposure with each patient has great potential to improve outcomes for all.

11

PROCESSING AND NEUROSCIENCE

Awareness of the importance of processing how patients experienced their imaginal and in vivo exposures—and how this affects treatment outcomes—has increased in the past several years. Indeed, in the revision of the prolonged exposure (PE) manual (Foa, Hembree, et al., 2019), additional information and clarification on how to implement this element was added on the basis of years of research and practice. Research on changes in trauma-related negative thoughts has shown us that greater confidence in one's ability to handle negative affect appears to be highly related to improvement in PE. When training providers in PE, it is key to discuss how therapists should make decisions about what to process based on where patients will gain the most therapeutic benefit. Often, this means focusing processing where patients will most increase their sense of competence, both at the time of the trauma and in the present.

Processing at the end of each session provides time to review current status and new insights, as well as to reduce the arousal that comes with active imaginal exposure, so that the patient leaves with new thoughts to consider and with a return to a more baseline level of affective arousal. Thus, the processing makes implicit learning explicit with focus on observing and discussing how the patient demonstrated tolerance for negative affect, reduction in negative affective activation (both within-session extinction and between-session

https://doi.org/10.1037/0000242-011
Retraining the Brain: Applied Neuroscience in Exposure Therapy for PTSD,
by S. A. M. Rauch and C. P. McLean

extinction), and showed competence at the time of the trauma and now. These connections add to the therapeutic context of safety learning and provide avenues for alterations in perceived control as well as facilitating changes in the brain and stress response systems associated with better function and response to PE (Bollini et al., 2004; Donadon et al., 2018; Norrholm et al., 2016; Price et al., 2013; Sripada & Rauch, 2015).

Although a more thorough review of all the steps and elements of processing can be found in the PE manual, it is important to note key points. First, processing is patient directed. This means that the therapist begins with those new insights and thoughts that the patient brings up related to the imaginal exposure. If the patient does not raise something, or the therapist believes the patient may be avoiding other important content, then the therapist may ask about other specific content but, in general, maintains a facilitation role rather than a leader role during processing. It is important to note that this is *not* a form of Socratic questioning or cognitive restructuring as may occur in cognitive processing therapy. In fact, the therapist need not get to an alternate thought by the end of the session. More often, such alternate thoughts will develop over the course of treatment. In PE, the aim of processing is for the patient to consider alternative ways to view the trauma and their reactions to it, as they continue to engage in imaginal exposure during treatment. Processing simply helps patients attend to and articulate these alternative perspectives so that they will become part of the new extinction memory or of a new version of the trauma memory. The therapist serves as a nonjudgmental sounding board for patients to explore what happened, how they reacted at the time, what that reaction said about them at the time, and what the current treatment says about them now. This chapter will apply theory and neuroscience research to the work that clinicians do during postexposure processing and focus on how to optimize outcomes and maintenance of gains.

MAKING IMPLICIT LEARNING EXPLICIT

Processing always begins with review of the exposure. In most cases, the processing occurs after imaginal exposure, when the patients first open their eyes and the therapist provides initial encouragement ("Great job today!"), and then probes about how they perceived the exposure. One goal of processing is to make the implicit learning that occurs with each session explicit. Neuroscience provides an excellent rationale for this in showing how extinction learning is reflected in top-down processes reducing fear expression (see Chapter 4; see also S. A. M. Rauch & Liberzon, 2016). There are many ways that new learning that occurs during imaginal exposure (extinction) may provide this top-down reduction in fear expression. One specific path would include that information in the extinction context that signals safety, as opposed to threat, allows the brain to turn off fear expression based on a safety context. As another example, specifically reviewing the reduction in distress that the patient experienced across sessions can also help to tamp down fear expression. In addition, inhibitory processes in extinction learning provide support for strengthening extinction learning through explicit learning (Craske et al., 2014). Rather than assuming that their patients see their progress (e.g., in subjective units of distress [SUDS] lowering within a session or between sessions), therapists take the time and effort to discuss the pattern and its meaning and discuss any pattern variations. If a patient did not show change, then discussion of *why* is important (e.g., no change may be due to new material, or because the patient generally shows reduction in SUDS more slowly, etc.). In this review, the therapist aims to reflect back all the ways that the patient approached the trauma memory, stayed with the emotions it brought up, and was able to cope. Similar review may be usefully focused on with in vivo exposure. Either way, the consistent message is that patients can approach their trauma memory and reminders, that feared outcomes do not occur, that approaching the trauma memory gets easier with repetition, and that they can handle it. As patients learn these key lessons, they will gain hope and a sense of self-efficacy that they can get back to living a full life by systematically approaching the trauma reminders that are fueling avoidance.

Another specific item to review in processing is *safety learning*. This refers to going back to specifically review imaginal and in vivo exposures that went well. The goal is to point out and reflect back to patients that when they engaged in specific activities, nothing bad happened, and they were safe. Discussions of to *what* patients attribute the positive outcome can help generalize the learning to new situations or point to new exposures that may be needed. For instance, if patients attribute their being safe when they went to the grocery store as due to going at midnight, the therapist can process as follows: (a) they previously avoided the store even at night so this is an accomplishment that can be built upon, and (b) the next in vivo should not be at midnight to ensure generalization to other times of day when the patient wants to shop.

FACILITATING CONTEXTUALIZATION OF PREVIOUS FEAR LEARNING

In addition to reflecting the changes in emotion connected to the trauma memory, processing takes time to explore whether anything changed with the trauma memory. This may be new information included or previous information that now seems incorrect or no longer relevant. Although there is no requirement for new information to be added, changes to the imaginal exposure narrative almost always occur over the course of PE. As discussed in Chapter 4 on imaging, contextual information is part of fear learning—especially relevant to fear learning in posttraumatic stress disorder (PTSD) because studies show that trauma-related fear learning becomes decontextualized (Garfinkel et al., 2014; Rougemont-Bücking et al., 2011). Decontextualized fear learning means that, instead of simply applying the lessons learned from trauma to that particular incident, they become defining experiences for the person applied across situations. For instance, rape survivors who could not fight off their attackers may think of themselves as generally weak people, rather than seeing themselves as victims of strong attackers who have an intent to harm. Often for patients with PTSD, avoidance of the memory means that they have not really gone back to the trauma to think through what happened, why it happened, and what the experience does (or does not) say about them as a person. This often means that they have not considered the trauma context in their judgments about themselves and others at the time of the trauma. Take, for example, the case of a combat veteran with PTSD from an incident where she shot a young Iraqi girl who approached her convoy. If this patient judges herself as a murderer and avoids her trauma memory, she does not get a chance to consider the combat context (e.g., orders from her superior, operational procedures for managing potential threats) in which she made a very difficult decision.

Processing provides an opportunity to consider all the relevant contextual factors that may have contributed to the trauma, as well as a chance to incorporate this contextual information into the new extinction memory created through imaginal exposure. The pieces of context that are important may differ for different patients, but if therapists focus on discussion of previously discounted elements of the trauma context that may have contributed to the trauma and its outcome, then patients can consider different views and adopt perspectives that allow for a sense of mastery and, even, an opportunity to make amends if they continue to feel responsible. For the combat veteran who shot the child, moving from a context in which she viewed herself as a monster who killed a child to a combat context in which she shot the child to protect the whole convoy allowed her to feel sad about her choice but also to let go of the guilt for her action. Such shifts can help trauma survivors with PTSD to feel more competent in their reactions at the time, as well as more able to handle difficult situations and emotions in the present.

The elements of context that may be most helpful in boosting therapeutic response through increased safety learning or perceived control and, thus, that clinicians should focus on and reflect back can include the following:

(a) things the patient did at the time of trauma that aided in survival of self or others, (b) previously discounted elements of the trauma context that may have contributed to the trauma occurring (e.g., a combat environment, having been drugged, etc.), and (c) new thoughts they have about themselves and the world as related to the trauma. For many patients, processing is where they come to new conclusions that shift how they view the traumatic event and their role. This does not mean putting on rose-colored glasses and pretending that everyone is a hero, but it does mean that therapists provide a nonjudgmental space for patients to explore their trauma memory once the affect connected to the memory is slightly less intense. This often results in patients being able to move on from the trauma and stop seeing it as the definition of the self anymore and instead, seeing survival and recovery as their accomplishment. Readers are referred to the new version of the PE manual as well as Smith et al. (2013; see also Foa, Hembree, et al., 2019) for additional discussion of how to process context.

REFLECTION

Reflection as a clinical tool in PE is one way that clinicians can improve outcomes tied to these processes. Although we are referring here to nondirective reflection, the PE therapist is guiding the patient in that they are choosing among the many possible directions that can be explored after imaginal exposure on the basis of how the patient answers open-ended questions, such as, "How was that for you today?," "What came up today that you think is important for us to discuss?," or "What was different for you today compared with last week?" All of those open-ended questions can then lead to discussion and exploration of the trauma memory. In so doing, the therapist continues to reflect back patients' new thoughts and allows plenty of time for the patients to sit with and consider them. Patients are not required to commit to new perspectives, only to consider them, continue to do exposures, and to revisit them at the next session. The therapist can use a stance of collaborative empiricism to consider the new perspectives. For example, the therapist can model curiosity and interest in the different possible perspectives, and the patient and therapist can explore them together, without the need to push the patient toward any single alternate perspective. This provides a "chipping away" process for unhelpful thoughts (e.g., "I am a monster for killing a child") to loosen their grip and allow new thoughts to be considered (e.g., "I was following orders and keeping my buddies safe"). The goal is not presenting the evidence and deciding on a new perspective but reflecting back any statements the patient makes that move in a therapeutic direction and then monitoring how that changes other thoughts and PTSD over time and sessions. Common follow-up processing probes include "Tell me more about that" or "I noticed that you said [some more helpful way of viewing the trauma], what does that mean to you?"

In conclusion, neuroscience provides solid direction for how to optimize processing in PE, particularly around making implicit learning explicit and facilitating contextualization of learning. Focusing on the role of extinction learning and inhibitory processes in extinction learning can assist therapists in allocating session time, with an eye toward maximizing patient gains and session efficiency. Extinction learning and inhibitory processes can suggest specific and efficient ways to incorporate critical information into the new extinction memories that are generated over the course of PE, allowing patients to experience increased competence and control over negative affect and boosting therapeutic efficacy.

PART **IV** FUTURE DIRECTIONS

12 AUGMENTATION OF PROLONGED EXPOSURE

The breadth, quantity, and quality of the evidence supporting the efficacy and effectiveness of prolonged exposure (PE) are arguably stronger than for any other posttraumatic stress disorder (PTSD) treatment. However, dropout from treatment and lack of clinically meaningful response are issues relevant to all PTSD treatments. An early study of civilian PE trials found that 25% to 45% of patients continued to meet diagnostic criteria for PTSD at the end of treatment (van Minnen et al., 2002), consistent with the range of rates reported more recently (e.g., 31%; Zoellner et al., 2019). Although diagnostic status is not a sensitive measure of treatment change, studies do not consistently report metrics of change, and those that do differ in how such change is operationalized. However, regardless of the exact percentage of patients, it is safe to say that there is at least an important minority of patients who do not benefit sufficiently from PE.

Further, approximately one third of patients drop out from treatment (ending treatment prior to what protocol considers a full dose; Bradley et al., 2005; Hembree et al., 2003; Kehle-Forbes et al., 2016). Recent research using massed protocols instead of weekly therapy has shown consistently high retention (e.g., Beidel, Frueh, et al., 2017; Beidel, Stout, et al., 2017; S. A. M. Rauch, Yasinski, et al., 2020) relative to weekly sessions, suggesting that the pace of weekly

https://doi.org/10.1037/0000242-012
Retraining the Brain: Applied Neuroscience in Exposure Therapy for PTSD,
by S. A. M. Rauch and C. P. McLean

treatment may not maximize therapeutic momentum or patient motivation. Indeed, in the first author's clinical experience, patients who completed massed protocols often reported that daily sessions were beneficial in keeping them in care and reported having previously tried PE or another PTSD treatment on a weekly basis but felt unable to return for additional sessions. Although dropout is not always an indicator of poor outcome (i.e., once patients have benefited there is less need to attend additional sessions; Szafranski et al., 2017), over-all it is associated with worse outcomes than treatment retention (Berke et al., 2019). As more research trials have been conducted in veteran and active-duty military populations, it has become clear that the efficacy of PE and other evidence-based PTSD treatments is somewhat attenuated in these groups relative to civilians, for reasons that are not yet clear (Steenkamp et al., 2015). Thus, despite the impressive track record of PE, there is room for improvement.

The efficacy ceiling for PE is not well understood and innovative research is needed to identify the processes that contribute to both nonresponse and dropout. There are a number of different methods that researchers have used to improve or augment PE, and these depend, in part, upon the specific goal. For example, some strategies aim to improve overall efficacy, such that all patients achieve better outcomes or achieve good outcomes more efficiently, whereas other strategies may focus on reducing dropout or identifying the subset of patients at risk for nonresponse or slow response and applying targeted strategies.

PSYCHOTHERAPY AUGMENTATION

Several studies have explored whether the effects of PE can be bolstered or augmented by incorporating additional psychotherapy techniques. Some of the very first trials of PE were psychotherapy augmentation studies. The logic being that if A and B are both efficacious, outcomes will be further improved if A and B are combined. However, in contrast to study hypotheses, neither stress inoculation therapy (Foa, Dancu, et al., 1999) nor cognitive therapy (Foa et al., 2005; Marks et al., 1998) were found to significantly augment PE. Similarly, Paunovic and Öst (2001) found that exposure therapy (imaginal and in vivo delivered sequentially) was not significantly different from a cognitive behavioral theraphy (CBT) program comprised of exposure, cognitive therapy, and breathing retraining. In contrast to this pattern, a study by Bryant, Moulds, et al. (2008) found that adding cognitive restructuring (CR) to the combination of in vivo and imaginal exposure did yield superior outcomes. However, postimaginal exposure processing was intentionally omitted from this trial, and, because processing likely overlaps with CR in terms of therapeutic mechanisms, the results of Bryant, Moulds, et al. did not suggest that CR enhances PE when provided per protocol.

In a dismantling study of cognitive processing therapy, Resick et al. (2008) compared the full protocol to each of its two primary components: cognitive therapy and written imaginal exposure ("written accounts" of the trauma). Exposure alone was similarly efficacious to the full protocol and to cognitive therapy on interviewer-assessed PTSD. Exposure alone was inferior to the full treatment on self-reported PTSD symptoms at posttreatment, but this difference was no longer significant at follow-up (Resick et al., 2008). Another trial compared traditional imaginal exposure with imaginal exposure plus imagery rescripting (Arntz et al., 2007). *Imagery rescripting* involves changing the traumatic imagery to "correct" the situation in fantasy to produce a more favorable outcome (Arntz & Weertman, 1999). For example, a patient may reimagine the trauma as though they had greater control and agency in the situation, such that a feeling of helplessness is replaced with a feeling of mastery. Results showed that imaginal exposure plus imagery rescripting was not superior to imaginal exposure alone, although the authors highlight a higher dropout rate in imaginal exposure alone (Arntz et al., 2007).

Studies have also investigated whether there is benefit in adding emotional or social skills training to exposure therapy programs. Beidel et al. (2011) found that adding social emotional group therapy to trauma management therapy, comprised of imaginal and in vivo exposure plus group social skills training, did not increase PTSD reduction compared with imaginal and in vivo exposure alone, but it did increase social activity. Bryant et al. (2013) found that preceding exposure therapy (imaginal and in vivo implemented sequentially) with skills training was superior to preceding it with supportive counseling. These studies indicate that adding skills training to exposure therapy is better than adding supportive counseling. Because these studies use most, but not all, components of PE and did not include a PE-only condition, it is difficult to draw conclusions about the value of adding skills training to standard PE.

A quantitative review of these additive psychotherapy studies showed that there is a small but statistically significant advantage for treatments comprised of exposure plus additional components compared with exposure alone on interviewer-assessed PTSD, but not for self-reported PTSD, loss of diagnosis, or rates of treatment dropout (Kehle-Forbes et al., 2013). Importantly, the differences on interviewer-assessed PTSD were not clinically significant (Bisson et al., 2007). Given the cost of additional training and obstacles involved in dissemination of multiple protocols, consideration of what additive interventions or augmentation provide clinically significant changes may represent a low threshold alteration dissemination.

PHARMACOTHERAPY AUGMENTATION

Another line of research tested whether adding serotonin reuptake inhibitors (SRIs), which are efficacious for treating PTSD on their own, can improve PE outcomes. Results of an early study were promising. Schneier et al. (2012) found that PE plus paroxetine was more efficacious than PE plus placebo in reducing PTSD severity. However, the additive benefits disappeared by follow-up. Subsequent studies have not found evidence that pharmacotherapy augments PE. Popiel et al. (2015) found no evidence supporting the addition of paroxetine to PE. A large trial by S. A. M. Rauch et al. (2019) found that PE plus sertraline, PE plus placebo, and sertraline plus enhanced medication management were all efficacious in reducing PTSD, with no significant differences across groups. Zoellner et al. (2019) also found no difference between similar conditions.

Among patients who did not respond to an initial course of PE, Simon et al. (2008) found that the addition of paroxetine yielded no increased benefit over continued PE alone. Using a similar design but targeting those who did not respond to an initial course of sertraline, Rothbaum et al. (2006) found that those randomized to PE experienced significantly greater reductions in PTSD than those randomized to ongoing sertraline, but only for patients who showed a partial response to sertraline during the initial treatment phase. Thus, in general, findings from RCTs combining PE with SRIs do not provide strong evidence to support the addition of pharmacotherapy overall.

PHARMACOLOGICAL AUGMENTATION OF EXTINCTION

Research has also sought to identify and test pharmacological agents that can augment the therapeutic learning processes that underlie successful exposure therapy. This work is based on evidence from basic research with animals that shows pharmacological augmentation of extinction learning and memory reconsolidation (e.g., Dębiec & Ledoux, 2004) and that has subsequently been translated to clinical populations. This line of research can be distinguished from pharmacotherapy augmentation in that the pharmacological agent is administered only as a supplement to exposure therapy sessions; the agent does not treat anxiety or PTSD in and of itself.

d-Cycloserine

Although the results of early studies of d-cycloserine (DCS) and other so-called cognitive enhancers with other anxiety disorder populations were positive, studies of DCS hypothesized to enhance extinction learning have not demonstrated a clear beneficial effect in PTSD. de Kleine et al. (2012) found that DCS, a partial N-methyl-D-aspartate (NMDA) receptor agonist, did not augment PE, although augmentation was observed among a subgroup of completers. A study testing a six-session program (four sessions of imaginal exposure DCS alone, i.e., not PE) found that, contrary to expectation, DCS was associated with worse outcomes relative to placebo (Litz et al., 2012). The results of a pilot randomized controlled trial (RCT) testing whether DCS augmented virtual reality exposure for PTSD were more promising (Difede et al., 2014). The results of this study showed a nonsignificant medium effect at posttreatment and a significant large effect at the 6-month follow-up. Thus, although findings are somewhat mixed, they are consistent with data across anxiety disorders showing only small effects for DCS over placebo (Mataix-Cols et al., 2017). A recent meta-analysis that aimed to examine the apparent decline in the efficacy of DCS over the past 14 years found that, across anxiety disorders, more DCS doses (up to nine) and administering DCS more than 60 minutes before exposures were associated with a significant augmentation effect (Rosenfield et al., 2019). Those procedures match those used by de Kleine et al. and Difede et al. (which showed limited support for DCS augmentation) but not Litz et al. (2012; which showed a negative effect of DCS), suggesting that this pattern may hold for PTSD specifically.

Hydrocortisone

Hydrocortisone is a synthetic glucocorticoid that mimics the effects of cortisol, which is released by the hypothalamic–pituitary–adrenal (HPA) axis in response to stress and has important effects on extinction learning and memory (for a review, see de Quervain et al., 2009). Hydrocortisone could potentially augment exposure therapy by enhancing the consolidation of extinction learning, or inhibiting retrieval of traumatic memories, or both. In an experimental study, Surís et al. (2010) found that veterans who were administered hydrocortisone after one exposure session (writing about traumatic memories) reported significantly lower PTSD avoidance and numbing symptoms when presented with a script based on the written exposure 1 week later, as compared with those who received placebo. However, this difference disappeared at the 1-month follow-up assessment. Building on the promising findings of a case report (Yehuda et al., 2010), a pilot RCT ($N = 24$) found that veterans who received PE plus hydrocortisone experienced greater reduction in PTSD symptoms than those who received placebo (Yehuda et al., 2015). This difference was accounted for by greater retention in PE among those who received hydrocortisone. The findings also indicated that those with elevated glucocorticoid responsiveness at pretreatment were more likely to respond to treatment. However, a study providing dexamethasone prior to virtual reality exposure therapy as a way to activate the HPA axis showed increased dropout and no augmentation of impact (Maples-Keller, Jovanovic, et al., 2019). Since dexamethasone inhibits endogenous cortisol release—rather than augmenting— it is unclear what this means for cortisol augmentation. In summary, there is some limited data supporting the use of hydrocortisone as a PE augmentation strategy, but further research is needed.

Propranolol

Propranolol is a synthetic β-adrenergic receptor blocker that has peripheral noradrenergic effects and central inhibitory effects on protein synthesis. Experimental research has found that propranolol affects memory reconsolidation, presumably because protein synthesis is required for memory consolidation, and propranolol is a protein synthesis inhibitor (for an overview, see Lonergan et al., 2012). To date, only one RCT (Brunet et al., 2008) has compared the effects of propranolol to placebo in the context of exposure. This trial ($N = 19$) examined the effects of propranolol administered after one 20-minute exposure session. Upon reexposure to the trauma script 1 week later, participants who had received propranolol showed lower heart rate and skin conductance than those who received placebo. However, data on the impact on PTSD symptoms were not reported. Three subsequent open trials ($Ns = 28, 7,$ and 7) have evaluated the potential of propranolol to enhance exposure therapy (Brunet et al., 2011). Although findings to date show promise, controlled trials that report the effects of propranolol on PTSD symptoms are needed.

Cannabinoids

A growing body of literature demonstrates that the endogenous cannabinoid system modulates neuronal activation during stressful and fearful situations (de Bitencourt et al., 2013; Gunduz-Cinar et al., 2013). This system has been implicated in the consolidation of fear and fear extinction memories, and it has been proposed that enhancing CB_1 transmission may facilitate fear extinction in humans. The nonselective CB_1/CB_2 ligand delta-9-tetrahydrocannabinol (THC) exerts its central effects through agonism of the CB_1 receptor. THC is the primary constituent of cannabis and is responsible for the subjective effects of marijuana (Wachtel et al., 2002). Building on promising animal research (e.g., Chhatwal et al., 2005; de Bitencourt et al., 2008; Marsicano et al., 2002), experimental fear conditioning studies have found mixed evidence that the pre-extinction administration of THC facilitates extinction of conditioned fear in humans. Findings are equivocal; some have found that THC facilitates recall of extinguished fear (Rabinak et al., 2013, 2018), whereas others (Hammoud et al., 2019; Klumpers et al., 2012; Rabinak et al., 2014) have found no advantage for THC over placebo on 1-week extinction recall, although there is some evidence for greater extinction retention after a 1-day delay. Moreover, Hammoud et al. (2019) found that THC was associated with significant amygdala and ventromedial prefrontal cortex (vmPFC) activation, consistent with the possibility of enhanced extinction learning and perhaps memory consolidation. Although there is growing evidence that THC modulates the underlying neural circuits involved in fear extinction in humans, future clinical trials with PTSD patients are needed to show whether cannabinoids might augment exposure therapy and are currently underway (C. A. Rabinak, personal communication, Fall 2020).

Oxytocin

The neuropeptide oxytocin has been considered a promising candidate for PE augmentation because of its ability to enhance prosocial cognition and behavior (thought to promote the therapeutic alliance) and extinction learning (see Olff et al., 2010). An early study by Pitman et al. (1993) found that a single dose of oxytocin did not reduce physiological reactivity during one session of exposure therapy for PTSD. A large ($N = 120$) RCT by van Zuiden et al. (2017) targeting the prevention of PTSD found that twice-daily doses of oxytocin for 8 days did not significantly attenuate the onset on PTSD compared with placebo among emergency department patients. However, among participants with elevated PTSD symptoms at baseline, those who received oxytocin showed greater reduction in symptoms over time than those who received placebo, suggesting some efficacy of oxytocin on existing PTSD but not on the prevention of new PTSD. The second RCT to date ($N = 17$; Flanagan et al., 2018) compared self-administered oxytocin versus placebo prior to each of 10 PE sessions. No differences emerged between groups at the end of treatment on either self-reported or clinician-administered PTSD scales. However, there was a modest effect favoring oxytocin in self-reported PTSD symptoms at PE Session 3, when imaginal exposures begin (and risk for treatment dropout is elevated), providing preliminary evidence for accelerated symptom reduction. Replication in larger samples is needed to determine whether oxytocin does accelerate PTSD recovery during PE. It is worth noting that there is also an extensive literature on the effects of oxytocin on withdrawal symptoms, craving, and self-administration among individuals with substance-use dependence (McRae-Clark et al., 2013), highlighting the potential therapeutic value of oxytocin for those with PTSD and comorbid substance dependence.

Methylene Blue

Methylene blue, methylthioninium chloride, is thought to augment learning by increasing oxygen consumption and available adenosine triphosphate (ATP) during memory consolidation (Rojas et al., 2012). In animal research, methylene blue has been found to improve memory consolidation (Callaway et al., 2002; Riha et al., 2005) and extinction learning (Gonzalez-Lima & Bruchey, 2004; Wrubel et al., 2007). One study in humans ($N = 23$) found evidence that methylene blue augments exposure therapy for claustrophobia for those with low postexposure distress (Telch et al., 2014). Zoellner et al. (2017) tested the effects of postexposure methylene blue versus placebo administration following six sessions of daily imaginal exposure. The results showed large clinical gains across both groups that did not differ across groups, although nonsignificant effect-size differences emerged at the 3-month follow-up for PTSD severity (small effect) and reliable change (medium effect). The methylene blue group showed a delayed initial response followed by accelerated recovery, which differed from the linear pattern of symptom reduction for the placebo group. It may be that methylene blue delayed gains by consolidating the distress experienced in initial exposures rather than extinction learning that occurs over repeated sessions. These preliminary findings point to the potential utility of using methylene blue to augment PE, as well as a need for replication that explores administering methylene blue only in the later sessions of PE.

Yohimbine

The alpha-2 adrenergic receptor antagonist yohimbine is thought to facilitate fear extinction by increasing noradrenergic activity (Singewald et al., 2015), which in turn increases exposure-related arousal, thereby improving treatment effects either by promoting emotional engagement (emotional processing theory) or maximizing expectancy violations (inhibitory learning theory). Building on mixed but promising findings from other anxiety-related disorders, to date, one RCT ($N = 26$) tested the potential augmentation effect of yohimbine on PE outcomes. Tuerk et al. (2018) found that one pretreatment dose of yohimbine significantly reduced trauma-cued heart rate reactivity (this was the primary outcome of the study) relative to placebo, although there were no differences in PTSD severity across groups. The results justify further evaluation of yohimbine as a PE augmentation strategy.

Ketamine

Ketamine has been traditionally used as an alternative to general anesthesia. It acts as an antagonist of the glutamate N-methyl-D-aspartate (NMDA) receptor (Rasmussen, 2015). Because high NMDA receptor activation has been implicated in PTSD development (McGhee et al., 2008) and because ketamine functions as an antagonist to the NMDA receptor, it has been proposed as a potential PTSD prevention and treatment strategy. Limited animal studies, case reports, and naturalistic studies suggest a possible link between ketamine and reduced PTSD-related symptoms (see Liriano et al., 2019). One proof-of-concept, randomized crossover study ($N = 41$) found that, compared with placebo, a single intravenous dose of ketamine was associated with significant reduction in PTSD symptoms 24 hours after infusion, but that there were no group differences 7 days postinfusion. To date, no studies have tested ketamine as a possible augmentation strategy in PTSD treatment. However, there is evidence that ketamine infusion leads to neurobiological changes that can enhance learning (see Duek et al., 2019), which suggests that it could enhance extinction learning in the context of PE. Future studies are needed to examine whether additional infusions provide greater long-term efficacy and whether adding ketamine to PE augments efficacy.

MDMA

MDMA (±3,4-methylenedioxymethamphetamine) is a substituted phenetylamine that binds and reverses monoamine transporters, causing the release of serotonin and, to a lesser extent, norepinephrine and dopamine. MDMA could potentially impact extinction learning through several mechanisms, including increased activity in the ventromedial prefrontal cortex (vmPFC) and decreased amygdala activity (Phelps et al., 2004), enhanced cortisol and norepinephrine levels, or increased oxytocin levels (Johansen & Krebs, 2009). To date only two studies have tested MDMA as an augmentation strategy in treating PTSD. A small trial ($N = 20$) by Mithoefer et al. (2011) found that MDMA was superior to pill placebo in reducing PTSD symptoms at posttreatment and from 17 to 74 months later (Mithoefer et al., 2013) among civilians who had failed a course of psychotherapy or pharmacotherapy for PTSD. Treatment in this study included two predrug sessions followed by four drug-enhanced 8- to 10-hour-long nondirective sessions (exposure to the traumatic experience occurred spontaneously) and then by four integration sessions to discuss the experiences of the enhanced sessions. A second pilot study ($N = 12$; Oehen et al., 2013), using a similar sample and protocol, also found evidence that MDMA was superior to placebo. Although the effects were attenuated relative to Mithoefer et al. (2011), it is important to note that because MDMA causes salient subjective effects, patients who receive placebo are not blind to treatment. In addition, the nondirective psychotherapy protocol used in the above studies is procedurally very different from standard exposure therapy and probably should not be considered exposure therapy. Studies that test the potential augmenting effect of MDMA on established exposure treatments are needed and underway (B. O. Rothbaum, personal communication, Fall 2020).

TRANSCRANIAL MAGNETIC STIMULATION

Repetitive transcranial magnetic stimulation (rTMS) is a noninvasive technique that aims to modulate cortical and subcortical function through rapidly changing electromagnetic fields generated by a coil of wire placed on the scalp. rTMS can be used to increase or decrease excitability in relatively focal areas, depending on the parameters of stimulation. Successful application of rTMS for treatment-resistant major depressive disorder has led researchers to evaluate its efficacy for PTSD, given the impairments in extinction learning recall observed in PTSD linked with hypoactivation of the prefrontal cortex (including medial and dorsolateral regions) and hyperactivation of the amygdala (S. L. Rauch et al., 2006). As a result, numerous trials have examined whether rTMS targeting the dorsolateral prefrontal cortex (dlPFC) may ameliorate PTSD or hyperarousal symptoms specifically. Several small trials ($Ns \leq 30$) found support for the use of rTMS as a stand-alone treatment for PTSD when administered in 10 sessions over 2 to 3 weeks to the right dlPFC (Boggio et al., 2010; H. Cohen et al., 2004; Nam et al., 2013; Watts et al., 2012). Other studies explored the application of rTMS as an augmentation strategy to determine whether stimulation to actively engaged, rather than passive, brain regions may be a more effective method of modifying dysfunctional brain circuitry. In a crossover design, Osuch et al. (2009; $N = 9$) found that graduated imaginal exposure to stressful events plus rTMS to the right dlPFC was associated with greater reductions in hyperarousal symptoms only (not significant) than imaginal exposure plus sham rTMS, with no differences on other PTSD outcomes. Focusing on the media prefrontal cortex, a pilot study ($N = 30$) by Isserles et al. (2013) tested deep TMS (DTMS) versus sham DTMS with 12 sessions of script-driven imagery and found that DTMS after imagery of traumatic experience led to a significant reduction in heart rate during exposure and intrusive symptoms and a trend for improvement in the total PTSD symptoms. In the only large RCT ($N = 103$) to date, Kozel et al. (2018) compared 12 sessions of cognitive processing therapy (CPT; including written accounts) with 30 minutes of either rTMS or sham rTMS to the right dlPFC prior to each session among veterans with PTSD. The findings were positive: rTMS was associated with significantly greater reductions in PTSD symptoms up to 6 months posttreatment with large ($d \geq 0.79$) effects relative to sham rTMS. In a subsequent small pilot ($N = 8$), veterans with PTSD were randomized to eight sessions of PE preceded by 30 minutes of sham rTMS or rTMS to the right dlPFC (Fryml et al., 2019). Reduction in interviewer-assessed PTSD symptoms was 15% greater for those who received rTMS than for those who did not. Additional research with sufficiently large sample sizes is needed to determine whether rTMS augments exposure therapy.

Theta-burst stimulation (TBS) is a novel transcranial magnetic stimulation (TMS) technique that involves repeated short bursts of high-frequency stimulation that can be administered intermittently (iTMS) or continuously. Translational models suggest that TBS can increase hippocampal activity (Capocchi et al., 1992), suggesting a possible role for enhancing memory consolidation of extinction learning. Also, because TBS is faster than rTMS, it may be more feasible to deliver, either as a stand-alone treatment or as a psychotherapy augmentation strategy. One study examined 10 days of sham-controlled iTBS followed by 10 unblinded sessions in 50 veterans with PTSD (Philip et al., 2019). Results showed nonsignificant medium effects favoring iTMS on self-reported PTSD, and significant differences on self-reported and interviewer-assessed PTSD at 1-month follow-up, which incorporated data from the unblinded phase. Given that most of the reductions in PTSD occurred early, future studies should examine the optimal duration of iTMS. The potential role of iTMS as an exposure therapy augmentation strategy should also be investigated.

Many have concluded that additional research examining dosing and timing of these more specific learning augmentation strategies (e.g., medications, TMS) is needed to see when and how to use such cognitive enhancers to help clarify their potential utility. Specifically, certain key conditions were not consistently controlled across previous studies, such as providing enhancers only after sessions where therapeutic learning occurred and ensuring that dosing occurred at a specific time interval prior to the imaginal exposure to allow enhancement mechanisms to be activated.

BEHAVIORAL AUGMENTATION

Exercise has documented antidepressive and anxiolytic effects that have made it useful as an intervention for depressive and anxiety disorders (Jayakody et al., 2014), including PTSD (Rosenbaum et al., 2015). Exercise may affect pathological anxiety through several mechanisms, including reduction of anxiety sensitivity, changes in serotonergic and endorphinergic systems, increased self-efficacy, or extinction learning related to exercise-induced exposure to physiological sensations (Asmundson et al., 2013). In addition, exercise has been found to increase brain-derived neurotrophic factor (BDNF) significantly, which is crucial for synaptic plasticity in brain regions that are critically involved in the consolidation of extinction learning (Andero & Ressler, 2012). Building on positive findings from an animal study showing that exercise increased extinction learning (Siette et al., 2014), Powers et al. (2015) evaluated exercise as a PE augmentation strategy in a small pilot trial ($N = 9$). Participants who completed 30 minutes of moderate-intensity treadmill exercise prior to each PE session showed elevated BDNF and greater reduction in PTSD symptoms relative to the PE-only condition, with large effects for both outcomes. On the basis of these preliminary findings, and the feasibility of implementing exercise into clinical care, further investigation into exercise-augmented exposure therapy is warranted. Including peers who have completed PE to assist with in vivo homework is a strategy that has been explored to minimize dropout from PE. Survey data suggest that approximately half of participants who drop out of PE report a greater likelihood of PE completion if they received in vivo social support and about a third of patients indicate that they would be willing to re-initiate treatment with peer support (Hernandez-Tejada et al., 2017). Indeed, a study of peer support found that about one third of those who dropped out of PE returned to treatment after being offered in vivo peer support (Hernandez-Tejada, Acierno, & Sánchez-Carracedo, 2020). An ongoing RCT is comparing in vivo peer support to general telephone support among 150 veterans who have indicated that they intend to drop out of PE (Hernandez-Tejada, Muzzy, et al., 2020). If successful, augmenting treatment with in vivo peer support could represent a new strategy to effectively minimize the rate of dropout from PE.

ALTERNATIVE MEDICINE APPROACHES

Needle acupuncture is hypothesized to help adults with PTSD by triggering neurological responses involving the autonomic nervous system, the prefrontal cortex, and several limbic structures in the brain involved in the pathophysiology of PTSD (Hollifield, 2011). One study found that adding acupuncture to usual PTSD care was associated with superior reduction of PTSD symptoms (Engel et al., 2014). Another study reported positive results for adding acupoint stimulation to exposure-based CBT among earthquake survivors (Y. Zhang et al., 2011), but inadequate descriptions of study methodology make its use difficult to interpret. At present, there is insufficient data on the potential efficacy, or information about possible mechanisms, of acupuncture as an exposure therapy augmentation strategy.

Biofeedback involves providing patients with feedback on real-time changes in physiological activity (i.e., heart rate variability, breathing). Breathing biofeedback has been evaluated as an adjunct to PE (implemented during imaginal exposure) in a small ($N = 8$) trial that found a nonsignificant trend for faster change in self-reported PTSD symptoms from baseline to 1 week post-treatment for those who received breathing biofeedback. The small sample and lack of follow-up limit the interpretability of the findings, but it should be noted that reducing physiological arousal during exposure runs counter to proposed mechanisms of action in exposure therapy and PE. For instance, one mechanism of PE requires activation of the memory, including emotions associated and remaining with those activated emotions, to see that nothing bad happens. Providing an intervention with the goal to reduce that activation is inconsistent with the overall message of exposure therapy that emotions are not harmful or dangerous to experience.

IDIOGRAPHIC APPROACHES

Idiographic approaches that identify *patient demographics* (e.g., gender, ethnic/racial groups) or *clinical characteristics* (e.g., trauma type, comorbidities), ideally those that are easily measured pretreatment, could be leveraged to make clinically useful predictions about which treatment a given patient is most likely to complete and benefit from (Imel et al., 2013). Unfortunately, most psychotherapy RCTs are not adequately powered for subgroup analyses that could determine which treatment works best for whom, so there is currently little evidence to guide clinicians on treatment selection. Some early work in this area has begun to identify univariate and multivariate models of patient factors that predict differential risk of dropout for PE. Specifically, Markowitz et al. (2015) found that comorbid depression was associated with elevated risk of dropout for PE relative to interpersonal therapy and that sexual trauma was associated with superior efficacy for interpersonal therapy relative to PE despite equivalent efficacy overall (Markowitz et al., 2017). Rizvi et al. (2009) found that for both PE and cognitive processing therapy (CPT), younger age, lower intelligence, and less education were associated with greater risk of dropout, whereas higher depression and guilt at pretreatment were associated with greater improvement in PTSD symptoms. This study also found that for PE specifically, women with higher anger at pretreatment were more likely to drop out and that older women in PE demonstrated the largest reductions in PTSD symptoms.

Although studies of single patient-level moderators of dropout and treatment response could inform clinical recommendations for treatment selection, if there are multiple moderators that are not strongly correlated with each other, it would be possible for a patient to present with a combination of characteristics that both indicate and contraindicate a given treatment (Z. D. Cohen & DeRubeis, 2018). Using machine-learning and bootstrapping methodologies to test whether and how a set of characteristics may combine to predict differential retention and engagement, Keefe et al. (2018) found that despite equivalent dropout rates between PE and CPT, patients who were assigned to their model-indicated treatment were significantly less likely to drop out than patients who were not. Significant moderators included in the model were childhood physical abuse, current relationship conflict, anger, and being a racial minority, which were associated with higher likelihood of dropout in PE than CPT.

Another promising line of research has focused on identifying biomarkers that are associated with PTSD treatment response. This work has found that changes to neuroendocrine systems seem to be linked with PTSD treatment response (S. A. M. Rauch, King, et al., 2015; Sageman & Brown, 2006). If individual differences in these neuroendocrine factors help account for the variability in response to PE, baseline differences could be used to predict the probability of achieving a good outcome with PE versus needing additional or alternate interventions and/or predict the estimated rate of recovery. Previous work has found that cortisol awakening response and increased cortisol reactivity in response to a brief personal trauma script at baseline predicted greater response to PE (S. A. M. Rauch, King, et al., 2015). In addition, lower salivary cortisol in response to a trauma-potentiated startle paradigm at baseline was also found to predict PTSD treatment (alprazolam plus virtual reality exposure therapy; Norrholm et al., 2016). Other work suggests that changes in the endogenous neuroactive steroid dehydroepiandrosterone (DHEA) are observed over the course of effective trauma-focused treatment (Olff et al., 2007). Elevations in the endogenous neuroactive steroid ALLO (allopregnanolone and pregnanolone) have been associated with lower anxiety in response to trauma-related stimuli (Rasmusson & Pineles, 2018), and elevations in DHEA in response to adrenocorticotropic hormone (ACTH) challenge have been associated with lower PTSD severity in women (Rasmusson et al., 2004). These preliminary findings suggest that ALLO and

DHEA, as well as markers of HPA axis function, may represent prognostic factors for PE response.

Further research on predictors and moderators of PE treatment is needed to develop treatment selection models that could increase efficacy or efficiency or reduce dropout by matching patients with interventions that they are most likely to benefit from.

13 NEW MODELS OF CARE DELIVERY

Based on neuroscience research and other research pointing to potential mechanisms of response to prolonged exposure (PE) as reviewed throughout this book, many are moving to new models of care to improve efficacy, retention, and speed of response. Some of the most relevant new models of PE are summarized in this chapter. Most studies of PE have implemented the protocol in once-weekly, 90-minute sessions, although some studies have done twice-weekly sessions (e.g., Foa, Dancu, et al., 1999; Resick et al., 2002; Rothbaum et al., 2006). The weekly session format is consistent with the practice standard in mental health for many disorders. At this pace, a typical course of PE (eight to 15 sessions) is from 2 to 4 months. However, when providers are unable to see patients weekly (e.g., due to large patient caseloads) or when patients occasionally miss sessions, treatment can last even longer, adversely affecting the momentum of therapeutic gains and making it difficult to attain the full dose of treatment. Indeed, many patients are unable to complete a full course of treatment (Imel et al., 2013), and longer courses of treatment are associated with higher dropout (Fernandez et al., 2015) and worse clinical outcomes relative to shorter treatments.

Almost all studies of PE have been implemented in specialty mental health clinics (an exception, Foa et al., 2005, was implemented in a community

https://doi.org/10.1037/0000242-013
Retraining the Brain: Applied Neuroscience in Exposure Therapy for PTSD,
by S. A. M. Rauch and C. P. McLean

clinic). Even in routine clinical practice, evidence-based practices (EBPs) such as PE are not routinely available in the community. Attending weekly appointments in specialty mental health clinics is challenging for many post-traumatic stress disorder (PTSD) patients. Common barriers to accessing this type of traditional PTSD treatment include the lack of available services, the need to travel significant distances to clinics, difficulty scheduling sessions during work hours (and/or coordinating child care), and fear of stigmatization associated with mental health problems (Morland et al., 2017). Among veterans, high demand for mental health services and staffing shortages may increase patient wait times and discourage treatment seeking (Hobfoll et al., 2016). Many PTSD patients are unwilling to follow through on a referral to specialty mental health services and, as such, do not get an opportunity to receive this treatment option. Furthermore, the significant commitment required for 90-minute sessions across many weeks can be an obstacle for patients with PTSD, who are often struggling with other life stressors. Studies evaluating novel methods of delivering PE, or exposure therapy more broadly, have expanded considerably in the past decade. Researchers are testing new delivery schedules, new adaptations, and using technology to implement new formats of exposure that hold promise in addressing barriers to standard care and increasing the reach of PE.

MASSED TREATMENT

Attending weekly sessions over multiple months is a challenge for many PTSD patients, and growing evidence suggests that more frequent sessions can lower dropout from treatment and accelerate recovery (Gutner et al., 2016). There has been considerable interest in modifying PE and other evidence-based psychotherapies for PTSD to be delivered in a condensed or "massed" format, in which sessions are delivered daily rather than weekly. This significantly reduces the overall length of treatment, which in turn can make it easier to complete a full dose of treatment, thereby optimizing the potential for a positive outcome. Massed treatment may also help to limit avoidance, which can interfere with treatment motivation and momentum, because patients experience reductions in PTSD symptoms more quickly and are in more frequent contact with their therapist, who can address avoidance promptly.

The first randomized controlled trial (RCT; Foa et al., 2018) to test PE in a massed format was conducted with active-duty military personnel at Fort Hood, Texas. Identifying effective massed treatment is particularly important in the military health system, because service members are often unable to attend weekly therapy sessions regularly due to military training schedules and job requirements. The large trial ($N = 366$) compared four study conditions: (a) 10 sessions of standard weekly PE delivered over 8 weeks (the first and last two sessions were conducted in the same week), (b) 10 sessions of weekly present-centered therapy (PCT) over 8 weeks, (c) 10 sessions of daily PE over 2 weeks, and (d) minimal contact control. The results showed that massed PE was superior to minimal contact control in reducing PTSD symptoms and non-inferior to standard spaced PE. Two weeks posttreatment, 45% of the massed PE participants had lost their PTSD diagnosis. Moreover, the dropout rate for massed PE was very low: only 13.6%, compared with 22.7% for spaced PE, although this difference did not reach statistical significance. Providing further support for the safety of massed PE, a secondary analysis (L. A. Brown et al., 2019) revealed that more participants in massed PE experienced a reliable improvement versus reliable exacerbation in suicide ideation compared with those in minimal contact control.

Another RCT of massed PE replicated and extended the results of Foa et al. (2018) with a modified 3-week massed PE protocol. Massed PE was com-pared with a more intensive massed PE protocol that included several different "enhancements." Enhancements included (a) imaginal exposure conducted gradually with the three most distressing traumatic events, (b) imaginal expo-sure homework completed in the clinic, (c) two additional feedback sessions completed each day for processing reactions to imaginal exposure and in vivo homework, and (d) three posttreatment booster sessions completed. Both treatment conditions were associated with large effects in reducing PTSD, with no significant differences between conditions at posttreatment. However, by the 6-month follow-up, interviewer-assessed PTSD symptoms showed more reduction in the massed PE condition than the unenhanced massed PE condi-tion. Although both forms of massed PE were effective, the intensive massed PE condition showed more maintenance of treatment gains. It is difficult to know why because the intensive condition included several differences from the stan-dard massed condition.

Massed PE was also found to be efficacious in an open trial among indi-viduals with PTSD related to multiple traumas and prior treatment attempts (L. Hendriks et al., 2018). In this protocol, PE was initially massed, and then subsequent sessions were spaced. Participants ($N = 73$) received 12 sessions total, with three sessions daily over 4 days followed by four weekly sessions. PTSD symptoms significantly decreased from baseline to posttreatment with large effect size. At the 6-month follow-up, 45% had lost their PTSD diagnosis on the basis of the Clinically Administered PTSD Scale (CAPS) assessment. There was no dropout during the massed phase and 5% during the spaced phase.

Massed PE is currently being implemented for post-9/11 veterans and service members through the Emory Healthcare Veterans Program. This 2-week program provides daily PE (one 90-minute individual session and one 120-minute group in vivo session) and clinically indicated adjunctive interventions. Effectiveness data ($N = 80$) revealed low dropout (4%); significant reduction in PTSD, depression, and neurobehavioral symptoms related to traumatic brain injury; and improved social function over 2 weeks, with 95% of participants reporting satisfaction with the program (S. A. M. Rauch et al., 2020b; Yasinski et al., 2018). A subsequent qualitative study focused on patient impressions of the massed protocol ($N = 25$) and revealed that participant reactions were more positive (51%) than negative (18%). Key identified benefits of massed PE were that the program structure limits distractions and avoidance and that experiencing rapid reductions in symptoms enhances motivation and engagement. Key identified drawbacks were the short-term discomfort of engaging in exposure and the program's demands in terms of effort and time.

Trauma management therapy (TMT) is a multicomponent treatment that includes individual exposure therapy plus group interventions that are delivered in an intensive, 3-week outpatient format (Beidel, Stout, et al., 2017). A large open trial ($N = 100$) tested massed TMT that included daily individual imaginal exposure using virtual reality, homework in vivo exposure, and group therapy for anger management, behavioral activation, and social skills (Beidel, Frueh, et al., 2017). Results showed large reductions in PTSD symptoms that were maintained at 6 months posttreatment with low (2%) dropout. In summary, although data are limited to date, it appears that massed PE/exposure therapy is comparably efficacious to spaced treatment, acceptable to patients, and associated with high treatment retention.

SHORTER SESSIONS

PE protocol calls for 90-minute therapy sessions to allow for enough time for prolonged imaginal exposure. However, the standard 90-minute PE session format constitutes a barrier to implementation in most mental health settings, which traditionally operate using a 60-minute session framework, corresponding to insurance billing codes. In addition, providers in many settings face pressures to meet high quotas for patient care (measured by relative value units [RVUs]), which, when combined with a large caseload of patients, make it difficult to see patients in 90-minute weekly therapy slots. Reducing PE sessions from 90 minutes to 60 minutes would remove a significant practical barrier to the adoption of PE.

Since PE was first developed, a robust literature related to extinction learning in animals has indicated that within-trial (session) fear reduction is not related to fear extinction (i.e., long-term fear reduction), suggesting that shortening exposure sessions may be feasible without reducing treatment efficacy. Data from human samples, as reviewed in Chapter 6 (on psychophysiological methods), also point to this feasibility. Within-session extinction is not reliably associated with treatment outcome. There are two studies to date that have examined this issue within the context of PTSD. In a nonrandomized study, van Minnen and Foa (2006; $N = 92$) found that 60-minute imaginal exposures (in 90-minute sessions) did not produce superior outcomes to 30-minute imaginal exposures (in 60-minute sessions). In a pilot RCT ($N = 39$), Nacasch et al. (2015) found that 20-minute imaginal exposures (during 60-minute sessions) were as effective as 40-minute imaginal exposures (during 90-minute sessions). Preliminary results of a noninferiority trial suggest that 60-minute PE sessions are noninferior to the standard 90-minute sessions in terms of both efficacy (reduction in PTSD symptoms) and efficiency (number of sessions needed to meet symptom-based criterion for recovery; Foa et al., 2020). The equivalency of shorter PE sessions promises to make it much easier for PE to be implemented, given the ubiquity of the 60-minute session framework.

ABBREVIATED TREATMENT

Another way to hasten recovery and lower dropout is to abbreviate exposure therapy such that fewer total sessions are required. Two protocols for brief exposure therapy for PTSD have been developed (see also PE for primary care in the next section; Cigrang et al., 2017). Developed for use in specialty mental health settings, *written exposure therapy* (WET; D. M. Sloan et al., 2012) is a brief exposure treatment that involves five weekly sessions of imaginal exposure via writing about the worst traumatic experience for 30 minutes. In WET, the therapist provides writing instructions and a postwriting check-in, but patients complete the writing exercise on their own, which significantly reduces direct face-to-face contact between therapist and patient. WET was found efficacious in reducing PTSD symptoms in a small pilot ($N = 7$) with veterans (D. M. Sloan et al., 2013) and in a controlled trial with civilians with PTSD ($N = 46$) related to a motor vehicle accident (D. M. Sloan et al., 2012, 2013). In a noninferiority trial ($N = 126$), WET (five sessions) was found noninferior to 12 weekly sessions of cognitive processing therapy (D. M. Sloan et al., 2018). Notably, WET has consistently demonstrated a very low dropout rate ($< 10\%$). On the basis of these data, WET is now recommended as a first-line treatment (VA/DoD, 2017).

Studies testing PE augmentation strategies often implement abbreviated versions of PE in order to lower the efficacy ceiling enough so that there is room to observe the hypothesized augmentation effect. It is worth noting that, although these protocols were not developed as stand-alone treatments, they have often demonstrated significant efficacy when combined with placebo. For example, the d-cycloserine (DCS) augmentation study by Litz et al. (2012) tested six weekly sessions with four sessions of imaginal exposure (with no homework and no in vivo), and both groups showed significant improvement with medium to large effects. The methylene blue study by Zoellner et al. (2017) implemented a protocol that was both abbreviated and massed, with six 50-minute daily sessions of imaginal exposure (no homework or in vivo). This treatment protocol led to significant reductions in PTSD, with about two thirds of patients losing their PTSD diagnosis at posttreatment (this increased to $\geq$ 87% by the 3-month follow-up).

As with massed treatments, shorter treatments seem to work well and minimize dropout compared with longer courses of treatment. In addition, these protocols appear to yield good outcomes despite requiring no between-session homework, which may increase patient acceptability. Future research is needed to determine who benefits from these shorter treatments versus who needs a longer course of treatment to achieve an optimal outcome.

PRIMARY CARE

EBP implementation is rare outside of specialty mental health clinics, and there are numerous barriers to accessing care in such settings, including the length of treatment. Most PTSD patients first present to primary care but often do not accept or follow through with referrals to specialty mental health (Possemato et al., 2011). Thus, delivering brief treatments for PTSD interventions in primary care could reduce barriers to accessing effective treatment.

PE for primary care (PE-PC) is a brief version of PE that was developed for implementation in primary care mental health settings (S. A. M. Rauch et al., 2017). The protocol includes four to six weekly, 30-minute sessions. Imaginal exposure is conducted via writing about the trauma and then reading the narrative, both in sessions and as homework, followed by emotional processing. Early findings from a pilot study ($N = 15$) found that PE-PC delivered in military treatment facilities was feasible and effective in reducing PTSD at posttreatment (Cigrang et al., 2011). A follow-up study ($N = 24$) reported that these gains were maintained 6 to 12 months posttreatment (Cigrang et al., 2015). To date, one RCT has evaluated PE-PC. Cigrang et al. (2017)

randomized service members ($N = 67$) to PE-PC or to a delayed-treatment minimal-contact control condition. At posttreatment, 40% had remitted from PTSD, and participants who received PE-PC showed significantly greater reductions in PTSD symptoms compared with minimal contact, with gains maintained through to 6 months posttreatment. Studies are underway in civilian primary care as well as by the Veteran Administration (VA) and Department of Defense (DoD). Training programs are currently underway in the Army, Air Force, and VA to train embedded mental·health providers in this intervention to greatly increase access to effective PTSD treatment. The intention of PE-PC is to provide quick access to an acceptable PTSD treatment that will provide a sufficient dose for many patients with PTSD presenting to primary care settings. For those who need additional care, facilitated referral to a full dose of PE or CPT in specialty care can be provided to meet their needs.

VIRTUAL REALITY

Virtual reality (VR) technology has been used to facilitate imaginal exposure using head-mounted computer simulations of sights, sounds, vibrations, and smells related to the individual's worst trauma memory. VR-facilitated imaginal exposure has been found to be efficacious in reducing PTSD severity as part of trauma management therapy in an open trial (Beidel, Frueh, et al., 2017). In augmentation trials, PE with VR-facilitated imaginal exposure has been found efficacious with and without the cognitive enhancer DCS (Difede et al., 2014; Rothbaum et al., 2014). A study comparing PE using VR to deliver imaginal exposure with PE using standard imaginal exposure found no differences between groups in reducing PTSD symptoms (Reger et al., 2016). A purported advantage of VR is that it helps the subset of patients who particularly struggle to engage with their trauma memory with sufficient detail and affective magnitude to benefit from exposure (Beidel et al., 2019). Although this hypothesis has not been tested directly, Reger et al. (2019) found no overall differences between VR-facilitated imaginal exposure and standard imaginal exposure in emotional activation as measured by subjective distress. Although the available evidence suggests that there is no added benefit for VR in terms of treatment outcomes, more research is needed to determine whether VR holds any advantages to standard imaginal exposure in terms of patient interest (i.e., promoting treatment seeking), emotional engagement/activation, or treatment retention. Future studies should examine if some PTSD patients benefit more from VR than standard PE.

TELEHEALTH

Considerable evidence now supports the efficacy of delivering PE via weekly telehealth videoconferencing. Because patients can access telehealth through a home computer or tablet, this model of care has potential to address numerous barriers to standard in-person, office-based treatment, including logistic barriers related to travel and stigma. A pilot study ($N = 12$) found that telehealth PE was feasible and effective in significantly reducing PTSD symptoms (Tuerk et al., 2010). A larger open trial ($N = 67$) also found that telehealth PE led to significant PTSD reductions, with a large effect size (Gros et al., 2011). Consistent with preliminary findings (Yuen et al., 2015), the final results of a noninferiority trial ($N = 132$) showed that 8 to 12 weeks of telehealth PE was noninferior to in-person PE in reducing PTSD symptoms, with treatment gains maintained through 6 months posttreatment (Acierno et al., 2017). Another noninferiority trial ($N = 132$) replicated this pattern, finding that telehealth PE was not inferior to standard in-person PE in reducing PTSD symptoms among veterans at posttreatment through to the 6-month follow-up. The most recent trial ($N = 175$) examined PE delivered in several ways: telehealth delivered at home, telehealth delivered at a VA office, and in-person at home (Morland et al., 2020). The results showed no significant differences between groups in the efficacy of PE in reducing PTSD symptoms. However, participants in the in-person at-home condition were less likely to drop out of treatment (presumably because it is difficult to avoid sessions when the therapist comes to your residence).

Telehealth PE appears to minimize much of the burden associated with standard in-person care without sacrificing efficacy. Indeed, telehealth PE is already being implemented widely in the VA health care system. Studies of treatments that combined telehealth with other new models of care (e.g., massed PE, written exposure therapy) are needed to identify further applications of telehealth. With the recent COVID-19 global pandemic, additional barriers to the provision to therapy via telehealth are being reduced daily, with the promise that this mode of care provision may remain in the forefront.

ᴇHEALTH

Delivering exposure therapy online through web-based eHealth treatments represents another innovative way to overcome barriers to in-person treatment. eHealth interventions have many of the benefits of telehealth in reducing logistical barriers to care seeking, and they have two additional advantages.

First, sessions do not need to be coordinated with a therapist's schedule, which provides greater flexibility in accessing treatment at a time and place of the patient's choosing. Second, because therapist contact is usually via email or telephone, eHealth treatments offer greater anonymity, which may minimize stigma-related concerns.

Two meta-analyses have found that web treatments for PTSD are efficacious compared with control condition with medium between-group effect sizes (Lewis et al., 2019; Simblett et al., 2017). Whereas most web treatments for PTSD focus on cognitive behavioral therapy (CBT), only a few have included exposure therapy. *Interapy* is a type of narrative exposure treatment that has been studied in various populations, including trauma-exposed samples, that involves structured writing exercises, including confronting the trauma memory followed by therapist feedback (Ruwaard et al., 2011). In a large trial ($N = 159$) of interapy in Arab patients with war-related PTSD, 10 twice-weekly interapy sessions were found to be significantly more efficacious in reducing self-reported PTSD symptoms compared with a waitlist control, with a large effect sized at posttreatment and 3-month follow-up (Knaevelsrud et al., 2015). A version of interapy adapted for military populations was also found to be efficacious in a small trial ($N = 34$) with veterans with PTSD as an adjunct to in-person treatment-as-usual (TAU) VA care (Krupnick et al., 2017). This study found that the online intervention Warriors Internet Recovery & EDucation (WIRED) was associated with greater reductions in self-reported PTSD symptoms, in particular hyperarousal symptoms, as compared with TAU, with a large between-group effect size at posttreatment and 24-week follow-up. However, this study had a high treatment dropout rate (75%) in the online treatment group, making it difficult to interpret the findings.

Ivarsson et al. (2014) used an RCT to compare an eight-session internet-delivered CBT ($N = 62$; in vivo and imaginal exposure via writing and reading of trauma narratives) with email therapist feedback to a minimal contact control. The results showed that the CBT condition was associated with significant reductions in self-reported PTSD symptoms with large between-group effects that were maintained through 1-year follow-up. Another RCT ($N = 52$) compared a similar eight-session online CBT program (in vivo and imaginal exposure via writing) with a delayed treatment control condition (Lewis et al., 2017). Online sessions were preceded with a 1-hour in-person session, and up to 30 minutes of in-person or telephone therapist contact was provided every 2 weeks. With an average therapist contact of only 2.5 hours, the online treatment was associated with significantly lower interviewer-assessed PTSD symptoms, with a large between-group effect size that was maintained at 1-month follow-up. In addition, a seven-session online CBT program, which included in vivo and imaginal exposure with therapist email and telephone support, was also found superior to waitlist in reducing interviewer-assessed PTSD (Spence et al., 2011).

An early trial of online CBT for PTSD represents the only study to date that has used an active online comparator. Litz et al. (2007) compared an online treatment that included in vivo exposure and imaginal exposure via writing with therapist feedback to an online supportive counseling condition that involved symptom monitoring, psychoeducation, and writing about current problems. Both treatments began with an in-person therapy session and included therapist support throughout. Participants who received the CBT condition showed a significantly greater decline in interviewer-assessed PTSD symptoms than the supportive counseling at posttreatment, although the difference was attenuated at the 3-month follow-up.

Note that none of these studies tested existing evidence-based treatments, such as PE, and none were compared with the standard format of psychotherapy: in-person delivery. To fill this gap, McLean et al. (2020) compared an online version of PE ("web-PE") to PCT delivered in-person in a small RCT ($N = 40$) with active-duty military personnel with PTSD. The results showed significant reductions in PTSD symptoms for both groups, with no significant differences between the two conditions on interviewer-assessed or self-reported PTSD at posttreatment and at 3- and 6-month follow-up, although effect sizes were larger for PCT ($d = 0.86$) than web-PE ($d = 0.58$). Gains were modest in both groups, and treatment dropout was higher in web-PE (47%) than in-person PCT (19%). Trial design required that participants be willing to do online or in-person therapy and complete multiple in-person assessments. This requirement may have biased the sample away from the target population for eHealth interventions: those who do not have access to in-person care or who are not able or willing to access this care. This hypothesis is supported by lower treatment credibility scores and higher dropout from web-PE compared with PCT. It is also consistent with the findings of a subsequent open trial of web-PE ($N = 34$) in which all participants were specifically seeking online treatment and all assessments were completed online. The results of the open trial showed that web-PE led to a significant reduction in self-reported PTSD symptoms with a large effect size ($d = 1.79$), although the dropout rate from treatment was similar (41%).

Overall, data from studies testing online exposure therapy programs are very promising, particularly considering the greater accessibility, cost effectiveness (because therapist time is significantly minimized), anonymity, and treatment fidelity that is afforded by the internet. A major challenge with online PTSD treatment is retention in treatment. The rates of dropout from treatment in the studies reviewed above range from 30% (Litz et al., 2007) to 75% (Krupnick et al., 2017). It may be that dropout rates are higher than for in-person treatment because accountability is lower and because ease of avoidance is greater in online treatment. Whereas most studies incorporate therapist oversight and feedback, an ongoing study is testing WET delivered online using peer support specialists in place of therapists (McLean et al., 2020). If efficacious, this could make eHealth exposure therapy even more cost effective and scalable.

mHEALTH

Mobile mental health apps ("mHealth") provide many of the advantages of online treatment with even greater accessibility. A key advantage of mHealth interventions is that they can be accessed at any time or place at relatively low costs (Hussain et al., 2015). They can also be used anonymously, which might be appealing to those who fear stigmatization (Andrade et al., 2014; Donker et al., 2013). Given the growing prevalence of smartphones globally and their ubiquity in daily life, mHealth interventions are a pinnacle of accessibility. However, although they are easy to access, they are also easy to ignore, presenting some unique challenges for researchers and app developers in this field.

Although mobile mental health apps have proliferated in recent years, PTSD still has some of the fewest mHealth interventions compared with other mental health conditions, such as anxiety or depression (Linardon et al., 2019). A recent review identified 12 mHealth interventions that were rated as good quality (Sander et al., 2020). Of these, 10 were self-guided and two were treatment companion apps, designed for use by patients engaged in in-person therapy. The only self-guided app for PTSD that has been empirically evaluated is PTSD Coach. PTSD Coach was found feasible and acceptable among 49 community trauma survivors with PTSD symptoms (Miner et al., 2016). In addition, this study found a small effect for reducing PTSD symptoms over a 1-month use period. A subsequent RCT ($N = 120$) found that 3 months of PTSD Coach was associated with greater improvements in self-reported PTSD, depression, and psychosocial functioning from baseline to follow-up compared with waitlist; however, there were no significant differences at posttreatment (Kuhn et al., 2017). This study also found that participants who received PTSD Coach were significantly more likely to achieve clinically significant PTSD symptom improvement than those in waitlist. Usage data indicated that participants used the app approximately once per week.

To determine whether adding human support could boost app engagement and outcomes, Tiet et al. (2019) evaluated PTSD Coach plus brief telephone support with paraprofessionals in 29 veterans with PTSD symptoms. Participants reported that phone support was helpful and that, among the 70%

who used PTSD Coach, more than 80% accessed the app a minimum of two to three times per week throughout the 3-month intervention period. The addition of clinician support was tested in a study of PTSD Coach in primary care (Possemato et al., 2016) that compared self-guided use alone to self-guided use plus four 20-minute sessions (in-person or telephone) that were focused on setting symptom reduction goals and helping the veteran to fully engage with the app content. Seven of the 10 veterans in the clinician-support condition versus three of the 10 veterans in the self-guided condition reported clinically significant improvements in PTSD symptoms. In addition, participants in the clinician-supported condition were more likely to access PTSD specialty care postintervention. Notably, PTSD Coach focuses on psychoeducation, symptom tracking, providing crisis support resources, and symptom management, but it does not include any exposure therapy tools. Thus, despite promising findings of web-based programs that use exposure techniques, there are currently no studies of mobile apps for PTSD that focus on exposure.

One exception is a pilot study of a mobile app called *Renew*, which focuses on in vivo exposure, imaginal exposure (via writing or using talk-to-text), and self-care (including relaxation and behavioral activation; M. Miller et al., 2020). Renew also includes a novel social support function designed to enlist friends and family to reinforce app engagement and provide accountability. The results of the pilot study demonstrate the initial feasibility and acceptability among 18 community trauma survivors, but future studies are needed to demonstrate whether Renew has clinical utility in reducing PTSD symptoms.

In blended-care models, mHealth interventions accompany in-person treatment to promote activity and symptom monitoring, mobile sensing, or automate therapy tasks (Ebert et al., 2018). PE Coach (Reger et al., 2013) is a patient-facing mobile app designed to support providers and patients engaged in in-person or telehealth-delivered PE. PE Coach includes psychoeducational content and features for patients to record their trauma narrative, complete and track in vivo exposure and imaginal exposure homework, practice breathing retraining, monitor PTSD symptom change, and schedule upcoming sessions. Uptake of PE Coach and positive perceptions among VA providers have been documented (Kuhn et al., 2015; Reger et al., 2017). Additional work is needed to determine whether PE Coach improves treatment retention, homework adherence, or outcomes.

CONCLUSION

Research on new models for delivering exposure therapy for PTSD has proliferated in the past decade. Massed treatments and abbreviated treatments have potential to accelerate recovery from PTSD, thereby minimizing suffering. Shorter treatments also present a more accessible treatment option for many patients. Delivering brief treatment in primary care is an important strategy to increase the reach of evidence-based practices to populations that would not otherwise access specialty PTSD care. Indeed, many individuals with PTSD never seek treatment or do so only after many years of suffering (Koenen et al., 2017; Zammit et al., 2018). Delivering imaginal exposure through virtual reality provides yet another option for patients with PTSD that may be particularly appealing to certain patients.

Barriers to receiving in-person PTSD treatment, such as distance to clinics, difficulty taking time off work for treatment, scheduling appointments, inadequate transportation, and concerns about stigma all work to deter access to in-person therapy. Telehealth-delivered PE circumvents many of these barriers with equal efficacy to in-person care. Telehealth does not, however, reduce therapist time. This is important because there are too few therapists trained in evidence-based practices such as PE to meet the demand for services. Indeed, the mental health system in the United States faces two interrelated challenges: (a) a lack of capacity of trained mental health providers, and (b) an inequitable geographic distribution of mental health services to rural areas. Mental health providers disproportionately reside in metropolitan areas (Andrilla et al., 2018), leaving rural areas with chronic shortages of PTSD providers (Hauenstein et al., 2006; Wallace et al., 2006). Known barriers to receiving in-person PTSD treatment are compounded in underserved rural settings.

Using eHealth and mHealth interventions to deliver treatment for PTSD is a promising way to address the capacity and equity challenges related to the delivery of PTSD services. The use of web treatments for PTSD has increased dramatically in the past decade (Simblett et al., 2017). RCTs have now demonstrated the efficacy of eHealth interventions for PTSD in numerous populations, including veterans with PTSD (Hobfoll et al., 2016; Krupnick et al., 2017). Given the ubiquity of smartphones, mHealth interventions have potential to deliver wide-reaching, convenient, evidence-based interventions for individuals with PTSD symptoms. However, much more research is needed to evaluate the utility of mHealth interventions in reducing PTSD symptoms. PTSD patients increasingly want to access mental health services independently, and they want to interact with providers and programs at a time and place of their choosing. Both eHealth and mHealth interventions are well positioned to accommodate this demand.

To meaningfully impact the public health burden of PTSD, flexible models of care delivery are needed to meet trauma survivors where they are, both geographically and psychologically (Morland et al., 2017). The novel approaches to delivering exposure therapy described above represent critical efforts toward this goal. When patient preferences for PTSD treatment are met, they tend to benefit more from treatment (Zoellner et al., 2019). Thus, the more options that are available to PTSD patients for receiving treatment, the more likely they will access an option that is well suited to their needs and preferences, improving both treatment reach and clinical outcomes.

Glossary

Terms that appear in this Glossary are either drawn directly or adapted with permission from the *APA Dictionary of Psychology* (2nd ed.), except where cited otherwise.

absolute power A summation of a specific band frequency (typically alpha, beta, delta, gamma, or theta) over a time period in electroencephalogram (EEG).

alleles An alternate form of a gene that occupies a given position on each of a pair of homologous chromosomes and is responsible for variation in inherited characteristics.

alpha band A summation of a specific band frequency in electroencephalogram (EEG) related to wakeful relaxation with eyes closed.

association studies Genetic studies using a case-control design to determine which variants (called *alleles*) are more common in people with the disorder (cases) as opposed to those without the disorder (controls).

candidate gene studies Studies that focus genetic association analysis on previously identified specific genes (from animal studies or previous human studies) to replicate in other samples.

connectivity analysis A method used in brain imaging and electroencephalogram (EEG) that examines how activations in the brain and its specific structures are correlated.

contingent negative variation (CNV) A slow event-related potential in electroencephalogram (EEG) arising in the interval between a warning signal (e.g., a light) and a signal that directs action (e.g., a specific word on the screen or a colored shape) and is indicative of readiness or expectancy of the action signal.

d-cycloserine (DCS) D-4-amino-3-isoxazolidone, partial agonist at the glycine recognition site of the glutamatergic NMDA receptor that enhances some types of learning.

differential diffusion Variations in size, white matter density, and so on in brain imaging.

error-related negativity An event-related potential in electroencephalogram (EEG) that follows commission or omission errors.

event-related potentials A specific pattern of electrical activity produced in the brain when a person is engaged in a cognitive act, such as discriminating one stimulus from another.

evoked potentials A specific pattern of electrical activity produced in a particular part of the nervous system, most often the brain, in response to external stimulation.

flanker task A task in which stimuli are assigned one of two responses and the participant is required to respond to the target stimulus when this is flanked by other stimuli. The stimuli are presented at a known location (such as fixation cross) and the flanking stimuli are associated with a response that is either the same as or different from that assigned to the target.

generalization The spread of effects of conditioning to stimuli that differ in certain aspects from the stimulus present during original conditioning.

genetic variance Differences in the observable characteristics (phenotype) of members of a population or species due to the spontaneous or environmentally induced genetic alterations or rearrangements.

go/no-go tasks Tasks denoting two stimuli discrimination procedures in which a particular action is reinforced in the presence of one stimulus (the go stimulus) and not reinforced in the presence of the other (the no-go stimulus). This task is used to examine processes involved in inhibition as well as error-related processes in both clinical assessment and research.

genome-wide studies A method of genetics examination that looks across the entire genome for variations related to a specific condition.

heart rate variability A measure of variation in time between heartbeats.

late positive potentials An event-related potential in electroencephalogram (EEG) reflecting attention to emotion.

mismatch negativity (MMN) An event-related potential in electroencephalogram (EEG) to an odd stimulus in a sequence of stimuli reflecting sensory processing of stimuli.

monozygotic twins Twins that develop from a single fertilized ovum that splits in the early stages after fertilization to produce two individuals with identical genes.

nadir The lowest point in the wave form in electroencephalogram (EEG).

noise In relationship to neuroscience research, noise is variance in the targeted measure that is not associated with the intended construct and may reflect other processes, errors in collection or processing, and the like.

N-methyl-D-aspartate (NMDA) An agonist that binds to a class of glutamate receptors that are both ligand-gated and voltage-sensitive.

peak The highest point in the wave form in electroencephalogram (EEG).

phenotype The observable characteristics of an individual, such as morphological or biochemical features and the presence or absence of a particular disease or condition.

polygenic risk scores (PRS) The measure of aggregate risk across genes in one sample that can be applied to future samples and may offer a more robust estimate of the genetic and gene-by-environment risks (Smoller, 2016).

power spectrum The total amplitude of brain activation in electroencephalogram (EEG) signal, usually within a frequency band.

recurrence risk ratio A comparison of the rates of disorders within family members to rates within unaffected families or to the population prevalence.

relative power The activation in a time period in one band in comparison with the power across all bands together.

Research Domain Criteria (RDoC) A conceptual framework for understanding mental health issues that examines phenomena across systems and levels of analysis.

sensitivity The probability that a given measure or test yields a positive diagnostic prediction for an individual who has the condition for which they are being tested.

single nucleotide polymorphisms (SNPs) The most common variation in genetic code, involving adenine, cytosine, guanine, and thymine nucleotides.

specificity The probability that a given measure or test yields a negative diagnostic prediction for an individual who does not have the condition for which they are being tested.

startle response An unlearned, rapid, reflex-like response to sudden, unexpected, and intense stimuli (e.g., loud noises, flashing lights). This response includes behaviors that serve a protective function, such as closing eyes, frowning by drawing the eyebrows together, and so forth.

transcranial magnetic stimulation A method used to apply magnetic stimulation to the brain for the purpose of changing brain activations, structure, and/or function.

ventral attention network A brain network that is involved in executive control related to the evaluation of stimuli salience and orientation.

References

Abdallah, C. G., Averill, C. L., Ramage, A. E., Averill, L. A., Goktas, S., Nemati, S., & Consortium, S. S. (2019). Salience network disruption in U.S. Army soldiers with posttraumatic stress disorder. *Chronic Stress, 3*. https://doi.org/10.1177/2470547019850467

Acierno, R., Knapp, R., Tuerk, P., Gilmore, A. K., Lejuez, C., Ruggiero, K., Muzzy, W., Egede, L., Hernandez-Tejada, M. A., & Foa, E. B. (2017). A non-inferiority trial of prolonged exposure for posttraumatic stress disorder: In person versus home-based telehealth. *Behaviour Research and Therapy, 89*, 57–65. https://doi.org/10.1016/j.brat.2016.11.009

Admon, R., Milad, M. R., & Hendler, T. (2013). A causal model of post-traumatic stress disorder: Disentangling predisposed from acquired neural abnormalities. *Trends in Cognitive Sciences, 17*(7), 337–347. https://doi.org/10.1016/j.tics.2013.05.005

Akiki, T. J., Averill, C. L., Wrocklage, K. M., Scott, J. C., Averill, L. A., Schweinsburg, B., Alexander-Bloch, A., Martini, B., Southwick, S. M., Krystal, J. H., & Abdallah, C. G. (2018). Default mode network abnormalities in posttraumatic stress disorder: A novel network-restricted topology approach. *NeuroImage, 176*, 489–498. https://doi.org/10.1016/j.neuroimage.2018.05.005

Almli, L. M., Mercer, K. B., Kerley, K., Feng, H., Bradley, B., Conneely, K. N., & Ressler, K. J. (2013). ADCYAP1R1 genotype associates with post-traumatic stress symptoms in highly traumatized African-American females. *American Journal of Medical Genetics. Part B, Neuropsychiatric Genetics, 162*(3), 262–272. https://doi.org/10.1002/ajmg.b.32145

American Psychiatric Association. (1987). *Diagnostic and statistical manual of mental disorders* (3rd ed.).

American Psychiatric Association. (2013). *Diagnostic and statistical manual of mental disorders* (5th ed.).

American Psychological Association. (2017). *Clinical practice guideline for the treatment of PTSD*. https://www.apa.org/ptsd-guideline/ptsd.pdf

Amir, N., Stafford, J., Freshman, M. S., & Foa, E. B. (1998). Relationship between trauma narratives and trauma pathology. *Journal of Traumatic Stress, 11*(2), 385–392. https://doi.org/10.1023/A:1024415523495

Anagnostaras, S. G., Gale, G. D., & Fanselow, M. S. (2001). Hippocampus and contextual fear conditioning: Recent controversies and advances. *Hippocampus, 11*(1), 8–17. https://doi.org/10.1002/1098–1063(2001)11:1<8::AID-HIPO1015>3.0.CO;2-7

Andero, R., & Ressler, K. J. (2012). Fear extinction and BDNF: Translating animal models of PTSD to the clinic. *Genes, Brain, & Behavior, 11*(5), 503–512. https://doi.org/10.1111/j.1601–183X.2012.00801.x

Andrade, L. H., Alonso, J., Mneimneh, Z., Wells, J. E., Al-Hamzawi, A., Borges, G., Bromet, E., Bruffaerts, R., de Girolamo, G., de Graaf, R., Florescu, S., Gureje, O., Hinkov, H. R., Hu, C., Huang, Y., Hwang, I., Jin, R., Karam, E. G., Kovess-Masfety, V., . . . Kessler, R. C. (2014). Barriers to mental health treatment: Results from the WHO World Mental Health surveys. *Psychological Medicine, 44*(6), 1303–1317. https://https://doi.org/10.1017/S0033291713001943

Andrilla, C. H. A., Patterson, D. G., Garberson, L. A., Coulthard, C., & Larson, E. H. (2018). Geographic variation in the supply of selected behavioral health providers. *American Journal of Preventive Medicine, 54*(6, Suppl. 3), S199–S207. https://doi.org/10.1016/j.amepre.2018.01.004

Arntz, A., Tiesema, M., & Kindt, M. (2007). Treatment of PTSD: A comparison of imaginal exposure with and without imagery rescripting. *Journal of Behavior Therapy and Experimental Psychiatry, 38*(4), 345–370. https://doi.org/10.1016/j.jbtep.2007.10.006

Arntz, A., & Weertman, A. (1999). Treatment of childhood memories: Theory and practice. *Behaviour Research and Therapy, 37*(8), 715–740. https://doi.org/10.1016/S0005-7967(98)00173-9

Asmundson, G. J., Fetzner, M. G., DeBoer, L. B., Powers, M. B., Otto, M. W., Smits, J. A. J. (2013). Let's get physical: A contemporary review of the anxiolytic effects of exercise for anxiety and its disorders. *Depression and Anxiety, 30*(4), 362–373.

Asukai, N., Saito, A., Tsuruta, N., Kishimoto, J., & Nishikawa, T. (2010). Efficacy of exposure therapy for Japanese patients with posttraumatic stress disorder due to mixed traumatic events: A randomized controlled study. *Journal of Traumatic Stress, 23*(6), 744–750. https://doi.org/10.1002/jts.20589

Back, S. E., Killeen, T., Badour, C. L., Flanagan, J. C., Allan, N. P., Ana, E. S., Lozano, B., Korte, K. J., Foa, E. B., & Brady, K. T. (2019). Concurrent treatment of substance use disorders and PTSD using prolonged exposure: A randomized clinical trial in military veterans. *Addictive Behaviors, 90*, 369–377. https://doi.org/10.1016/j.addbeh.2018.11.032

Baker, A., Mystkowski, J., Culver, N., Yi, R., Mortazavi, A., & Craske, M. G. (2010). Does habituation matter? Emotional processing theory and exposure therapy for acrophobia. *Behaviour Research and Therapy, 48*(11), 1139–1143. https://doi.org/10.1016/j.brat.2010.07.009

Baker, J. F., Cates, M. E., & Luthin, D. R. (2017). D-cycloserine in the treatment of post-traumatic stress disorder. *Mental Health Clinician, 7*(2), 88–94. https://doi.org/10.9740/mhc.2017.03.088

Bangel, K. A., van Buschbach, S., Smit, D. J. A., Mazaheri, A., & Olff, M. (2017). Aberrant brain response after auditory deviance in PTSD compared to trauma controls: An EEG study. *Scientific Reports, 7*(1), 16596. https://doi.org/10.1038/s41598-017-16669-8

Bauer, M. R., Ruef, A. M., Pineles, S. L., Japuntich, S. J., Macklin, M. L., Lasko, N. B., & Orr, S. P. (2013). Psychophysiological assessment of PTSD: A potential research domain criteria construct. *Psychological Assessment, 25*(3), 1037–1043. https://doi.org/10.1037/a0033432

Beck, A. T. (2009). *Depression: Causes and treatment.* University of Pennsylvania Press. https://doi.org/10.9783/9780812290882

Beck, A. T., Rush, A. J., Shaw, B. F., & Emergy, G. (1979). *Cognitive therapy of depression.* Basic Books.

Becker, J. V., Skinner, L. J., Abel, G. G., Axelrod, R., & Cichon, J. (1984). Sexual problems of sexual assault survivors. *Women & Health, 9*(4), 5–20. https://doi.org/10.1300/J013v09n04_02

Beckham, J. C., Vrana, S. R., May, J. G., Gustafson, D. J., & Smith, G. R. (1990). Emotional processing and fear measurement synchrony as indicators of treatment outcome in fear of flying. *Journal of Behavior Therapy and Experimental Psychiatry, 21*(3), 153–162. https://doi.org/10.1016/0005-7916(90)90002-3

Bedard-Gilligan, M., Zoellner, L. A., & Feeny, N. C. (2017). Is trauma memory special? Trauma narrative fragmentation in PTSD: Effects of treatment and response. *Clinical Psychological Science, 5*(2), 212–225. https://doi.org/10.1177/2167702616676581

Beidel, D. C., Frueh, B. C., Neer, S. M., Bowers, C. A., Trachik, B., Uhde, T. W., & Grubaugh, A. (2019). Trauma management therapy with virtual-reality augmented exposure therapy for combat-related PTSD: A randomized controlled trial. *Journal of Anxiety Disorders, 61*, 64–74. https://doi.org/10.1016/j.janxdis.2017.08.005

Beidel, D. C., Frueh, B. C., Neer, S. M., & Lejuez, C. W. (2017). The efficacy of trauma management therapy: A controlled pilot investigation of a three-week intensive outpatient program for combat-related PTSD. *Journal of Anxiety Disorders, 50*, 23–32. https://doi.org/10.1016/j.janxdis.2017.05.001

Beidel, D. C., Frueh, B. C., Uhde, T. W., Wong, N., & Mentrikoski, J. M. (2011). Multicomponent behavioral treatment for chronic combat-related posttraumatic stress disorder: A randomized controlled trial. *Journal of Anxiety Disorders, 25*(2), 224–231. https://doi.org/10.1016/j.janxdis.2010.09.006

Beidel, D. C., Stout, J. W., Neer, S. M., Frueh, B. C., & Lejuez, C. (2017). An intensive outpatient treatment program for combat-related PTSD: Trauma management therapy. *Bulletin of the Menninger Clinic, 81*(2), 107–122. https://doi.org/10.1521/bumc.2017.81.2.107

Benuto, L. T., Bennett, N. M., & Casas, J. B. (2020). Minority participation in randomized controlled trials for prolonged exposure therapy: A systematic review of the literature. *Journal of Traumatic Stress, 33*(4). https://doi.org/10.1002/jts.22539

Berke, D. S., Kline, N. K., Wachen, J. S., McLean, C. P., Yarvis, J. S., Mintz, J., Young-McCaughan, S., Peterson, A. L., Foa, E., Resick, P. A., Litz, B. T., & the STRONG STAR Consortium. (2019). Predictors of attendance and dropout in three randomized controlled trials of PTSD treatment for active duty service members. *Behaviour Research and Therapy, 118*, 7–17. https://doi.org/10.1016/j.brat.2019.03.003

Binder, E. B. (2009). The role of FKBP5, a co-chaperone of the glucocorticoid receptor in the pathogenesis and therapy of affective and anxiety disorders. *Psychoneuroenocrinology, 34*(Suppl. 1), S186–S195. https://doi.org/10.1016/j.psyneuen.2009.05.021

Birkett, M. A. (2011). The Trier Social Stress Test protocol for inducing psychological stress. *Journal of Visualized Experiments, 3238*(56), 3238. https://doi.org/10.3791/3238

Bisson, J. I., Ehlers, A., Matthews, R., Pilling, S., Richards, D., & Turner, S. (2007). Psychological treatments for chronic post-traumatic stress disorder: Systematic review and meta-analysis. *British Journal of Psychiatry, 190*, 97–104. https://doi.org/10.1192/bjp.bp.106.021402

Bluett, E. J., Zoellner, L. A., & Feeny, N. C. (2014). Does change in distress matter? Mechanisms of change in prolonged exposure for PTSD. *Journal of Behavior Therapy and Experimental Psychiatry, 45*(1), 97–104. https://doi.org/10.1016/j.jbtep.2013.09.003

Boggio, P. S., Rocha, M., Oliveira, M. O., Fecteau, S., Cohen, R. B., Campanhã, C., Ferreira-Santos, E., Meleiro, A., Corchs, F., Zaghi, S., Pascual-Leone, A., & Fregni, F. (2010). Noninvasive brain stimulation with high-frequency and low-intensity repetitive transcranial magnetic stimulation treatment for posttraumatic stress disorder. *Journal of Clinical Psychology, 71*(8), 992–999.

Bollini, A. M., Walker, E. F., Hamann, S., & Kestler, L. (2004). The influence of perceived control and locus of control on the cortisol and subjective responses to stress. *Biological Psychology, 67*(3), 245–260. https://doi.org/10.1016/j.biopsycho.2003.11.002

Borah, E. V., Wright, E. Ç., Donahue, D. A., Cedillos, E. M., Riggs, D. S., Isler, W. C., & Peterson, A. L. (2013). Implementation outcomes of military provider training in cognitive processing therapy and prolonged exposure therapy for post-traumatic stress disorder. *Military Medicine, 178*(9), 939–944. https://doi.org/10.7205/MILMED-D-13-00072

Borkovec, T. D., & Sides, J. K. (1979). Critical procedural variables related to the physiological effects of progressive relaxation: A review. *Behavorial Research and Therapy, 17*(2), 119–125. https://doi.org/10.1016/0005-7967(79)90020-2

Boudewyns, P., & Hyer, L. (1990). Physiological response to combat memories and preliminary treatment outcome in Vietnam veteran PTSD patients treated with direct therapeutic exposure. *Behavior Therapy, 21*(1), 63–87. https://doi.org/10.1016/S0005-7894(05)80189-3

Bouton, M. E. (1993). Context, time, and memory retrieval in the interference paradigms of Pavlovian learning. *Psychological Bulletin, 114*, 80–99. https://doi.org/10.1037/0033-2909.114.1.80

Bouton, M. E., & Swartzentruber, D. (1991). Sources of relapse after extinction in Pavlovian and instrumental learning. *Clinical Psychology Review, 11*(2), 123–140. https://doi.org/10.1016/0272-7358(91)90091-8

Bradley, R., Greene, J., Russ, E., Dutra, L., & Westen, D. (2005). A multidimensional meta-analysis of psychotherapy for PTSD. *American Journal of Psychiatry, 162*, 214–227. https://doi.org/10.1176/appi.ajp.162.2.214

Breslau, N., Reboussin, B. A., Anthony, J. C., & Storr, C. L. (2005). The structure of posttraumatic stress disorder: Latent class analysis in 2 community samples. *Archives of General Psychiatry, 62*(12), 1343–1351. https://doi.org/10.1001/archpsyc.62.12.1343

Britton, J. C., Phan, K. L., Taylor, S. F., Fig, L. M., & Liberzon, I. (2005). Corticolimbic blood flow in posttraumatic stress disorder during script-driven imagery. *Biological Psychiatry, 57*(8), 832–840. https://doi.org/10.1016/j.biopsych.2004.12.025

Brown, L. A., McLean, C. P., Zang, Y., Zandberg, L., Mintz, J., Yarvis, J. S., Litz, B. T., Peterson, A. L., Bryan, C. J., Fina, B., Petersen, J., Dondanville, K. A., Roache, J. D., Young-McCaughan, S., Foa, E. B., & the STRONG STAR Consortium. (2019). Does prolonged exposure increase suicide risk? Results from an active duty military sample. *Behaviour Research and Therapy, 118*, 87–93. https://doi.org/10.1016/j.brat.2019.04.003

Brown, V. M., LaBar, K. S., Haswell, C. C., Gold, A. L., McCarthy, G., Morey, R. A., & the Mid-Atlantic MIRECC Workgroup. (2014). Altered resting-state functional connectivity of basolateral and centromedial amygdala complexes in posttraumatic stress disorder. *Neuropsychopharmacology, 39*(2), 351–359. https://doi.org/10.1038/npp.2013.197

Brunet, A., Orr, S. P., Tremblay, J., Robertson, K., Nader, K., & Pitman, R. K. (2008). Effect of post-retrieval propranolol on psychophysiologic responding during subsequent script-driven traumatic imagery in post-traumatic stress disorder. *Journal of Psychiatric Research, 42*(6), 503–506. https://doi.org/10.1016/j.jpsychires.2007.05.006

Brunet, A., Poundja, J., Tremblay, J., Bui, E., Thomas, E., Orr, S. P., Azzoug, A., Birmes, P., & Pitman, R. K. (2011). Trauma reactivation under the influence of propranolol decreases posttraumatic stress symptoms and disorder: 3 open-label trials. *Journal of Clinical Psychopharmacology, 31*(4), 547–550. https://doi.org/10.1097/JCP.0b013e318222f360

Bryant, R. A., Felmingham, K., Kemp, A., Das, P., Hughes, G., Peduto, A., & Williams, L. (2008). Amygdala and ventral anterior cingulate activation predicts treatment response to cognitive behaviour therapy for post-traumatic stress disorder. *Psychological Medicine, 38*(4), 555–561. https://doi.org/10.1017/S0033291707002231

Bryant, R. A., Mastrodomenico, J., Hopwood, S., Kenny, L., Cahill, C., Kandris, E., & Taylor, K. (2013). Augmenting cognitive behaviour therapy for post-traumatic stress disorder with emotion tolerance training: A randomized controlled trial. *Psychological Medicine, 43*(10), 2153–2160. https://doi.org/10.1017/S0033291713000068

Bryant, R. A., Moulds, M. L., Guthrie, R. M., Dang, S. T., Mastrodomenico, J., Nixon, R. D., Felmingham, K. L., Hopwood, S., & Creamer, M. (2008). A randomized controlled trial of exposure therapy and cognitive restructuring for posttraumatic stress disorder. *Journal of Consulting and Clinical Psychology, 76*(4), 695–703. https://doi.org/10.1037/a0012616

Bryant, R. A., Moulds, M. L., Guthrie, R. M., Dang, S. T., & Nixon, R. D. V. (2003). Imaginal exposure alone and imaginal exposure with cognitive restructuring in treatment of posttraumatic stress disorder. *Journal of Consulting and Clinical Psychology, 71*(4), 706–712. https://doi.org/10.1037/0022–006X.71.4.706

Bryant-Davis, T., & Ocampo, C. (2005). Racist incident–based trauma. *Counseling Psychologist, 33*(4), 479–500. https://doi.org/10.1177/0011000005276465

Buck, N., Kindt, M., Hout, V. D., Steens, L., & Linders, C. (2006). Perceptual memory representations and memory fragmentation as predictors of post-trauma symptoms. *Behavioural and Cognitive Psychotherapy, 35*(3), 259–272. https://doi.org/10.1017/S1352465806003468

Butt, M., Espinal, E., Aupperle, R. L., Nikulina, V., & Stewart, J. L. (2019). The electrical aftermath: Brain signals of posttraumatic stress disorder filtered through a clinical lens. *Frontiers in Psychiatry, 10*, 368. https://doi.org/10.3389/fpsyt.2019.00368

Cahill, S. P., & Foa, E. B. (2007). Psychological theories of PTSD. In M. J. Friedman, T. M. Keane, & P. A. Resick (Eds.), *Handbook of PTSD: Science and practice* (pp. 55–77). Guilford Press.

Cahill, S. P., Rauch, S. A., Hembree, E. A., & Foa, E. B. (2003). Effect of cognitive-behavioral treatments for PTSD on anger. *Journal of Cognitive Psychotherapy, 17*(2), 113–131.

Cahill, S. P., Rothbaum, B. O., Resick, P. A., & Follette, V. (2009). Cognitive-behavioral therapy for adults. In E. B. Foa, T. M. Keane, M. J. Friedman, and J. A. Cohen (Eds.), *Effective treatments for PTSD: Practice guidelines from the International Society for Traumatic Stress Studies* (2nd ed., pp. 139–222). Guilford Press.

Callaway, N. L., Riha, P. D., Wrubel, K. M., McCollum, D., & Gonzalez-Lima, F. (2002). Methylene blue restores spatial memory retention impaired by an inhibitor of cytochrome oxidase in rats. *Neuroscience Letters, 332*(2), 83–86. https://doi.org/10.1016/S0304-3940(02)00827-3

Campbell, A. A., Wisco, B. E., Silvia, P. J., & Gay, N. G. (2019). Resting respiratory sinus arrhythmia and posttraumatic stress disorder: A meta-analysis. *Biological Psychology, 144*, 125–135. https://doi.org/10.1016/j.biopsycho.2019.02.005

Capocchi, G., Zampolini, M., & Larson, J. (1992). Theta burst stimulation is optimal for induction of LTP at both apical and basal dendritic synapses on hippocampal CA1 neurons. *Brain Research, 591*, 332–336. https://doi.org/10.1016/0006-8993(92)91715-Q

Carlson, M., Endlsey, M., Motley, D., Shawahin, L. N., & Williams, M. T. (2018). Addressing the impact of racism on veterans of color: A race-based stress and trauma intervention. *Psychology of Violence, 8*(6), 748–762. https://doi.org/10.1037/vio0000221

Carson, M. A., Paulus, L. A., Lasko, N. B., Metzger, L. J., Wolfe, J., Orr, S. P., & Pitman, R. K. (2000). Psychophysiologic assessment of posttraumatic stress disorder in Vietnam nurse veterans who witnessed injury or death. *Journal of Consulting and Clinical Psychology, 68*(5), 890–897. https://doi.org/10.1037/0022-006X.68.5.890

Carter, R. T. (2007). Racism and psychological and emotional injury: Recognizing and assessing race-based traumatic stress. *Counseling Psychologist, 35*(1), 13–105. https://doi.org/10.1177/0011000006292033

Castro-Chapman, P. L., Orr, S. P., Berg, J., Pineles, S. L., Yanson, J., & Salomon, K. (2018). Heart rate reactivity to trauma-related imagery as a measure of PTSD symptom severity: Examining a new cohort of veterans. *Psychiatry Research, 261*, 574–580. https://doi.org/10.1016/j.psychres.2018.01.024

Celec, P., Ostatníková, D., & Hodosy, J. (2015). On the effects of testosterone on brain behavioral functions. *Frontiers in Neuroscience, 9*, 12–12. https://doi.org/10.3389/fnins.2015.00012

Chaplin, E. W., & Levine, B. A. (1981). The effects of total exposure duration and inter-rupted versus continuous exposure in flooding therapy. *Behavior Therapy, 12*(3), 360–368. https://doi.org/10.1016/S0005-7894(81)80124-4

Charquero-Ballester, M., Kleim, B., Vidaurre, D., Ruff, C., Stark, E., Tuulari, J. J., & Ehlers, A. (2020). Effective psychological treatment for PTSD changes the dynamics of specific large-scale brain networks. *bioRxiv*, 2020.2001.2007.891986. https://doi.org/10.1101/2020.01.07.891986

Chhatwal, J. P., Davis, M., Maguschak, K. A., & Ressler, K. J. (2005). Enhancing canna-binoid neurotransmission augments the extinction of conditioned fear. *Neuropsy-chopharmacology, 30*, 516–524. https://doi.org/10.1038/sj.npp.1300655

Cigrang, J. A., Rauch, S. A., Avila, L. L., Bryan, C. J., Goodie, J. L., Hryshko-Mullen, A., & Peterson, A. L. (2011). Treatment of active-duty military with PTSD in primary care: Early findings. *Psychological Services, 8*(2), 104–113. https://doi.org/10.1037/a0022740

Cigrang, J. A., Rauch, S. A. M., Mintz, J., Brundige, A., Avila, L. L., Bryan, C. J., Goodie, J. L., Peterson, A. L., & the STRONG STAR Consortium. (2015). Treatment of active duty military with PTSD in primary care: A follow-up report. *Journal of Anxiety Dis-orders, 36*, 110–114. https://doi.org/10.1016/j.janxdis.2015.10.003

Cigrang, J. A., Rauch, S. A., Mintz, J., Brundige, A. R., Mitchell, J. A., Najera, E., Litz, B. T., Young-McCaughan, S., Roache, J. D., Hembree, E. A., Goodie, J. L., Sonnek, S. M., Peterson, A. L., & the STRONG STAR Consortium. (2017). Moving effective treatment for posttraumatic stress disorder to primary care: A randomized con-trolled trial with active duty military. *Families, Systems & Health, 35*(4), 450–462. https://doi.org/10.1037/fsh0000315

Cloitre, M., Petkova, E., Wang, J., & Lu, F. (2012). An examination of the influence of a sequential treatment on the course and impact of dissociation among women with PTSD related to childhood abuse. *Depression and Anxiety, 29*(8), 709–717.

Cloitre, M., Stovall-McClough, K. C., Nooner, K., Zorbas, P., Cherry, S., Jackson, C. L., Gan, W., & Petkova, E. (2010). Treatment for PTSD related to childhood abuse: A randomized controlled trial. *American Journal of Psychiatry, 167*(8), 915–924. https://doi.org/10.1176/appi.ajp.2010.09081247

Coffey, S. F., Schumacher, J. A., Nosen, E., Littlefield, A. K., Henslee, A. M., Lappen, A., & Stasiewicz, P. R. (2016). Trauma-focused exposure therapy for chronic posttrau-matic stress disorder in alcohol and drug dependent patients: A randomized con-trolled trial. *Psychology of Addictive Behaviors, 30*(7), 778–790. https://doi.org/10.1037/adb0000201

Cohen, H., Kaplan, Z., Kotler, M., Kouperman, I., Moisa, R., & Grisaru, N. (2004). Repetitive transcranial magnetic stimulation of the right dorsolateral prefrontal cortex in posttraumatic stress disorder: A double-blind, placebo-controlled study. *American Journal of Psychiatry, 161*(3), 515–524. https://doi.org/10.1176/appi.ajp.161.3.515

Cohen, Z. D., & DeRubeis, R. J. (2018). Treatment selection in depression. *Annual Review of Clinical Psychology, 14*, 209–236. Advance online publication. https://doi.org/10.1146/annurev-clinpsy-050817-084746

Cooper, A. A., Clifton, E. G., & Feeny, N. C. (2017). An empirical review of potential mediators and mechanisms of prolonged exposure therapy. *Clinical Psychology Review, 56*, 106–121. https://doi.org/10.1016/j.cpr.2017.07.003

Cooper, A. A., Zoellner, L. A., Roy-Byrne, P., Mavissakalian, M. R. F., & Feeny, N. C. (2017). Do changes in trauma-related beliefs predict PTSD symptom improvement in prolonged exposure and sertraline? *Journal of Consulting and Clinical Psychology, 85*(9), 873–882. https://doi.org/10.1037/ccp0000220

Cooper, N., & Clum, G. (1989). Imaginal flooding as a supplementary treatment for PTSD in combat veterans: A controlled study. *Behavior Therapy, 20*(3), 381–391. https://doi.org/10.1016/S0005-7894(89)80057-7

Costanzo, M., Jovanovic, T., Norrholm, S. D., Ndiongue, R., Reinhardt, B., & Roy, M. J. (2016). Psychophysiological investigation of combat veterans with subthreshold post-traumatic stress disorder symptoms. *Military Medicine, 181*(8), 793–802. https://doi.org/10.7205/MILMED-D-14-00671

Courtois, C. A., Sonis, J., Brown, L. S., Cook, J., Fairbank, J. A., Friedman, M., & Schulz, P. (2017). *Clinical practice guidelines for the treatment of posttraumatic stress disorder (PTSD) in adults*. American Psychological Association. https://www.apa.org/ptsd-guideline/

Craske, M. G., Hermans, D., & Vervliet, B. (2018). State-of-the-art and future directions for extinction as a translational model for fear and anxiety. *Philosophical Transactions of the Royal Society B: Biological Sciences, 373*(1742), 20170025.

Craske, M. G., Kircanski, K., Zelikowsky, M., Mystkowski, J., Chowdhury, N., & Baker, A. (2008). Optimizing inhibitory learning during exposure therapy. *Behaviour Research and Therapy, 46*, 5–27. https://doi.org/10.1016/j.brat.2007.10.003

Craske, M. G., & Mystkowski, J. L. (2006). *Exposure therapy and extinction: Clinical studies*. https://doi.org/10.1037/11474-011

Craske, M. G., & Rachman, S. J. (1987). Return of fear: Perceived skill and heart rate responsivity. *British Journal of Clinical Psychology, 26*(3), 187–199. https://doi.org/10.1111/j.2044-8260.1987.tb01346.x

Craske, M. G., Treanor, M., Conway, C. C., Zbozinek, T., & Vervliet, B. (2014). Maximizing exposure therapy: An inhibitory learning approach. *Behaviour Research and Therapy, 58*, 10–23. https://doi.org/10.1016/j.brat.2014.04.006

Culver, N. C., Stoyanova, M., & Craske, M. G. (2011). Clinical relevance of retrieval cues for attenuating context renewal of fear. *Journal of Anxiety Disorders, 25*(2), 284–292. https://doi.org/10.1016/j.janxdis.2010.10.002

Culver, N. C., Stoyanova, M., & Craske, M. G. (2012). Emotional variability and sustained arousal during exposure. *Journal of Behavior Therapy and Experimental Psychiatry, 43*(2), 787–793. https://doi.org/10.1016/j.jbtep.2011.10.009

Dębiec, J., & Ledoux, J. E. (2004). Disruption of reconsolidation but not consolidation of auditory fear conditioning by noradrenergic blockade in the amygdala. *Neuroscience, 129*(2), 267–272. https://doi.org/10.1016/j.neuroscience.2004.08.018

de Bitencourt, R. M., Pamplona, F. A., & Takahashi, R. N. (2008). Facilitation of contextual fear memory extinction and anti-anxiogenic effects of AM404 and cannabidiol in conditioned rats. *European Neuropsychopharmacology, 18*(12), 849–859. https://doi.org/10.1016/j.euroneuro.2008.07.001

de Bitencourt, R. M., Pamplona, F. A., & Takahashi, R. N. (2013). A current overview of cannabinoids and glucocorticoids in facilitating extinction of aversive memories: Potential extinction enhancers. *Neuropharmacology, 64*, 389–395. https://doi.org/10.1016/j.neuropharm.2012.05.039

de Kleine, R. A., Hendriks, G.-J., Kusters, W. J. C., Broekman, T. G., & van Minnen, A. (2012). A randomized placebo-controlled trial of D-cycloserine to enhance exposure therapy for posttraumatic stress disorder. *Biological Psychiatry, 71*(11), 962–968. https://doi.org/10.1016/j.biopsych.2012.02.033

de Kleine, R. A., Smits, J. A., Hendriks, G. J., Becker, E. S., & van Minnen, A. (2015). Extinction learning as a moderator of d-cycloserine efficacy for enhancing exposure therapy in posttraumatic stress disorder. *Journal of Anxiety Disorders, 34*, 63–67.

de Quervain, D. J., Aerni, A., Schelling, G., & Roozendaal, B. (2009). Glucocorticoids and the regulation of memory in health and disease. *Frontiers in Neuroendocrinology, 30*(3), 358–370.

Dickerson, S. S., & Kemeny, M. E. (2004). Acute stressors and cortisol responses: A theoretical integration and synthesis of laboratory research. *Psychological Bulletin, 130*(3), 355–391.

Difede, J., Cukor, J., Wyka, K., Olden, M., Hoffman, H., Lee, F. S., & Altemus, M. (2014). D-cycloserine augmentation of exposure therapy for post-traumatic stress disorder: A pilot randomized clinical trial. *Neuropsychopharmacology, 39*(5), 1052–1058. https://doi.org/10.1038/npp.2013.317

Difede, J., Malta, L. S., Best, S., Henn-Haase, C., Metzler, T., Bryant, R., & Marmar, C. (2007). A randomized controlled clinical treatment trial for World Trade Center attack-related PTSD in disaster workers. *Journal of Nervous and Mental Disease, 195*(10), 861–865. https://doi.org/10.1097/NMD.0b013e3181568612

DiGangi, J., Guffanti, G., McLaughlin, K. A., & Koenen, K. C. (2013). Considering trauma exposure in the context of genetics studies of posttraumatic stress disorder: A systematic review. *Biology of Mood & Anxiety Disorders, 3*(1), 2–2. https://doi.org/10.1186/2045-5380-3-2

Dohle, G. R., Smit, M., & Weber, R. F. (2003). Androgens and male fertility. *World Journal of Urology, 21*(5), 341–345. https://doi.org/10.1007/s00345–003–0365–9

Dollard, J., & Muiller, N. (1950). *Personality and psychotherapy: An analysis in terms of learning, thinking, and culture.* McGraw-Hill.

Donadon, M. F., Martin-Santos, R., & Osório, F. L. (2018). The associations between oxytocin and trauma in humans: A systematic review. *Frontiers in Pharmacology, 9*, 154–154. https://doi.org/10.3389/fphar.2018.00154

Donker, T., Petrie, K., Proudfoot, J., Clarke, J., Birch, M. R., & Christensen, H. (2013). Smartphones for smarter delivery of mental health programs: A systematic review. *Journal of Medical Internet Research, 15*(11), e247. https://doi.org/10.2196/jmir.2791

Dour, H. J., Wiley, J. F., Roy-Byrne, P., Stein, M. B., Sullivan, G., Sherbourne, C. D., Bystritsky, A., Rose, R. D., & Craske, M. G. (2014). Perceived social support mediates anxiety and depressive symptom changes following primary care intervention. *Depression and Anxiety, 31*(5), 436–442. https://doi.org/10.1002/da.22216

Duek, O., Kelmendi, B., Pietrzak, R. H., & Harpaz-Rotem, I. (2019). Augmenting the treatment of PTSD with ketamine—A review. *Current Treatment Options in Psychiatry, 6*(2), 143–153. https://doi.org/10.1007/s40501-019-00172-0

Duncan, L. E., Ratanatharathorn, A., Aiello, A. E., Almli, L. M., Amstadter, A. B., Ashley-Koch, A. E., Baker, D. G., Beckham, J. C., Bierut, L. J., Bisson, J., Bradley, B., Chen, C. Y., Dalvie, S., Farrer, L. A., Galea, S., Garrett, M. E., Gelernter, J. E., Guffanti, G., Hauser, M. A., . . . Koenen, K. C. (2018). Largest GWAS of PTSD (N=20070) yields genetic overlap with schizophrenia and sex differences in heritability. *Molecular Psychiatry, 23*(3), 666–673. https://doi.org/10.1038/mp.2017.77

Duval, E. R., Sheynin, J., King, A. P., Phan, K. L., Simon, N. M., Martis, B., Porter, K. E., Norman, S. B., Liberzon, I., & Rauch, S. A. M. (2020). Neural function during emotion processing and modulation associated with treatment response in a randomized clinical trial for posttraumatic stress disorder. *Depression and Anxiety, 37*(7), 670–681. https://doi.org/10.1002/da.23022

Ebert, D. D., Van Daele, T., Nordgreen, T., Karekla, M., Compare, A., Zarbo, C., & Jensen, K. L. (2018). Internet- and mobile-based psychological interventions: Applications, efficacy, and potential for improving mental health. *European Psychologist, 23,* 167–187. https://doi.org/10.1027/1016–9040/a000318

Ehlers, A., & Clark, D. M. (2000). A cognitive model of posttraumatic stress disorder. *Behaviour Research and Therapy, 38*(4), 319–345. https://doi.org/10.1016/S0005-7967(99)00123-0

Ehlers, A., Clark, D. M., Hackmann, A., McManus, F., Fennell, M., Herbert, C., & Mayou, R. (2003). A randomized controlled trial of cognitive therapy, a self-help booklet, and repeated assessments as early interventions for posttraumatic stress disorder. *Archives of General Psychiatry, 60*(10), 1024–1032. https://doi.org/10.1001/archpsyc.60.10.1024

Eiden, L. E. (2013). Neuropeptide-catecholamine interactions in stress. *Advances in Pharmacology, 68,* 399–404.

Ellis, A. (1977). Rational-emotive therapy: Research data that supports the clinical and personality hypotheses of RET and other modes of cognitive-behavior therapy. *Counseling Psychologist, 7*(1), 2–42. https://doi.org/10.1177/001100007700700102

Engel, C. C., Cordova, E. H., Benedek, D. M., Liu, X., Gore, K. L., Goertz, C., Freed, M. C., Crawford, C., Jonas, W. B., & Ursano, R. J. (2014). Randomized effectiveness trial of a brief course of acupuncture for posttraumatic stress disorder. *Medical Care, 52*(12, Suppl. 5), S57–S64. https://doi.org/10.1097/mlr.0000000000000237

Eriksen, B. A., & Eriksen, C. W. (1974). Effects of noise letters upon the identification of a target letter in a nonsearch task. *Perception & Psychophysics, 16*(1), 143–149. https://doi.org/10.3758/BF03203267

Etkin, A., Maron-Katz, A., Wu, W., Fonzo, G. A., Huemer, J., Vértes, P. E., Patenaude, B., Richiardi, J., Goodkind, M. S., Keller, C. J., Ramos-Cejudo, J., Zaiko, Y. V., Peng, K. K., Shpigel, E., Longwell, P., Toll, R. T., Thompson, A., Zack, S., Gonzalez, B., . . . O'Hara, R. (2019). Using fMRI connectivity to define a treatment-resistant form of post-traumatic stress disorder. *Science Translational Medicine, 11*(486), eaal3236. Advance online publication. https://doi.org/10.1126/scitranslmed.aal3236

Etkin, A., & Wager, T. D. (2007). Functional neuroimaging of anxiety: A meta-analysis of emotional processing in PTSD, social anxiety disorder, and specific phobia. *American Journal of Psychiatry, 164*(10), 1476–1488. https://doi.org/10.1176/appi.ajp.2007.07030504

Familoni, B. O., Gregor, K. L., Dodson, T. S., Krzywicki, A. T., Lowery, B. N., Jr., Orr, S. P., Suvak, M. K., & Rasmusson, A. M. (2016). Sweat pore reactivity as a surrogate measure of sympathetic nervous system activity in trauma-exposed individuals with and without posttraumatic stress disorder. *Psychophysiology, 53*(9), 1417–1428. https://doi.org/10.1111/psyp.12681

Fani, N., Tone, E. B., Phifer, J., Norrholm, S. D., Bradley, B., Ressler, K. J., Kamkwalala, A., & Jovanovic, T. (2012). Attention bias toward threat is associated with exaggerated fear expression and impaired extinction in PTSD. *Psychological Medicine, 42*(3), 533–543. https://doi.org/10.1017/S0033291711001565

Feeny, N. C., Zoellner, L. A., & Foa, E. B. (2002). Treatment outcome for chronic PTSD among female assault victims with borderline personality characteristics: A preliminary examination. *Journal of Personality Disorders, 16*(1), 30–40.

Fernandez, E., Salem, D., Swift, J. K., & Ramtahal, N. (2015). Meta-analysis of dropout from cognitive behavioral therapy: Magnitude, timing, and moderators. *Journal of Consulting and Clinical Psychology, 83*(6), 1108–1122. https://doi.org/10.1037/ccp0000044

Fitzgerald, J. M., Gorka, S. M., Kujawa, A., DiGangi, J. A., Proescher, E., Greenstein, J. E., Aase, D. M., Schroth, C., Afshar, K., Kennedy, A. E., Hajcak, G., & Phan, K. L. (2018). Neural indices of emotional reactivity and regulation predict course of PTSD symptoms in combat-exposed veterans. *Progress in Neuro-Psychopharmacology & Biological Psychiatry, 82*, 255–262. https://doi.org/10.1016/j.pnpbp.2017.11.005

Flanagan, J. C., Sippel, L. M., Wahlquist, A., Moran-Santa Maria, M. M., & Back, S. E. (2018). Augmenting prolonged exposure therapy for PTSD with intranasal oxytocin: A randomized, placebo-controlled pilot trial. *Journal of Psychiatric Research, 98*, 64–69. https://doi.org/10.1016/j.jpsychires.2017.12.014

Foa, E. B., Acierno, R., Muzzy, W., Rosenfield, D., Bredemeier, K. (2020, October 20–21). *90-minute versus 60-minute sessions of prolonged exposure for the treatment of PTSD* [Plenary presentation]. San Antonio Combat PTSD Conference, San Antonio, TX, United States.

Foa, E., & Cahill, S. P. (2001). Emotional processing in psychological therapies. In Neil J. Smelser and Paul B. Baltes (Eds.), *International encyclopedia of the social and behavioral sciences* (pp. 12363–12369). Pergamon.

Foa, E. B., Dancu, C. V., Hembree, E. A., Jaycox, L. H., Meadows, E. A., & Street, G. P. (1999). A comparison of exposure therapy, stress inoculation training, and their combination for reducing posttraumatic stress disorder in female assault victims. *Journal of Consulting and Clinical Psychology, 67*(2), 194–200. https://doi.org/10.1037/0022–006X.67.2.194

Foa, E. B., Ehlers, A., Clark, D. M., Tolin, D. F., & Orsillo, S. M. (1999). The posttraumatic cognitions inventory (PTCI): Development and validation. *Psychological Assessment, 11*(3), 303–314. https://doi.org/10.1037/1040–3590.11.3.303

Foa, E. B., Grayson, J. B., Steketee, G. S., Doppelt, H. G., Turner, R. M., & Latimer, P. R. (1983). Success and failure in the behavioral treatment of obsessive-compulsives. *Journal of Consulting and Clinical Psychology, 51*(2), 287–297. https://doi.org/10.1037/0022-006X.51.2.287

Foa, E. B., Gillihan, S. J., & Bryant, R. A. (2013). Challenges and successes in dissemination of evidence-based treatments for posttraumatic stress: Lessons learned from prolonged exposure therapy for PTSD. *Psychological Science in the Public Interest, 14*(2), 65–111. https://doi.org/10.1177/1529100612468841

Foa, E. B., Hembree, E. A., Cahill, S. P., Rauch, S. A. M., Riggs, D. S., Feeny, N. C., & Yadin, E. (2005). Randomized trial of prolonged exposure for posttraumatic stress disorder with and without cognitive restructuring: Outcome at academic and community clinics. *Journal of Consulting and Clinical Psychology*, *73*(5), 953–964. https://doi.org/10.1037/0022–006X.73.5.953

Foa, E. B., Hembree, E. A., & Rothbaum, B. O. (2007). *Prolonged exposure therapy for PTSD: Emotional processing of traumatic experiences—Therapist guide*. Oxford University Press. https://doi.org/10.1093/med:psych/9780195308501.001.0001

Foa, E. B., Hembree, E. A., Rothbaum, B. O., & Rauch, S. A. M. (2019). *Prolonged exposure therapy for PTSD: Emotional processing of traumatic experiences—Therapist guide* (2nd ed.). Oxford University Press. https://doi.org/10.1093/med-psych/9780190926939.001.0001

Foa, E. B., Huppert, J. D., & Cahill, S. P. (2006). Emotional processing theory: An update. In B. O. Rothbaum (Ed.), *Pathological anxiety: Emotional processing in etiology and treatment* (pp. 3–24). Guilford Press.

Foa, E. B., & Jaycox, L. H. (1999). Cognitive-behavioral theory and treatment of posttraumatic stress disorders. In D. Spiegel (Ed.), *Efficacy and cost-effectiveness of psychotherapy* (pp. 23–61). American Psychiatric Press.

Foa, E. B., & Kozak, M. J. (1985). Treatment of anxiety disorders: Implications for psychopathology. In A. H. Tuma & J. D. Maser (Eds.), *Anxiety and the anxiety disorders* (pp. 421–452). Lawrence Erlbaum Associates, Inc.

Foa, E. B., & Kozak, M. J. (1986). Emotional processing of fear: Exposure to corrective information. *Psychological Bulletin*, *99*, 20–35. https://doi.org/10.1037/0033–2909.99.1.20

Foa, E. B., & McLean, C. P. (2016). The efficacy of exposure therapy for anxiety-related disorders and its underlying mechanisms: The case of OCD and PTSD. *Annual Review of Clinical Psychology*, *12*, 1–28. https://doi.org/10.1146/annurev-clinpsy-021815-093533

Foa, E. B., McLean, C. P., Zang, Y., Rosenfield, D., Yadin, E., Yarvis, J. S., Mintz, J., Young-McCaughan, S., Borah, E. V., Dondanville, K. A., Fina, B. A., Hall-Clark, B. N., Lichner, T., Litz, B. T., Roache, J., Wright, E. C., Peterson, A. L., & the STRONG STAR Consortium. (2018). Effect of prolonged exposure therapy delivered over 2 weeks vs 8 weeks vs present-centered therapy on PTSD symptom severity in military personnel: A randomized clinical trial. *Journal of the American Medical Association*, *319*(4), 354–364. https://doi.org/10.1001/jama.2017.21242

Foa, E. B., & McNally, R. J. (1995). Mechanisms of change in exposure therapy. In R. M. Rapee (Ed.), *Current controversies in the anxiety disorders* (pp. 329–343). Guilford Press.

Foa, E. B., Molnar, C., & Cashman, L. (1995). Change in rape narratives during exposure therapy for posttraumatic stress disorder. *Journal of Traumatic Stress*, *8*(4), 675–690. https://doi.org/10.1002/jts.2490080409

Foa, E. B., & Rauch, S. A. M. (2004). Cognitive changes during prolonged exposure versus prolonged exposure plus cognitive restructuring in female assault survivors with posttraumatic stress disorder. *Journal of Consulting and Clinical Psychology*, *72*(5), 879–884. https://doi.org/10.1037/0022–006X.72.5.879

Foa, E. B., & Riggs, D. S. (1993). Post-traumatic stress disorder in rape victims. In J. M. Oldham, A. B. Riba, & A. Tasman (Eds.), *Annual review of psychiatry* (Vol. 12, pp. 273–303). American Psychiatric Association.

Foa, E. B., Riggs, D. S., Massie, E. D., & Yarczower, M. (1995). The impact of fear activation and anger on the efficacy of exposure treatment for posttraumatic stress disorder. *Behavior Therapy*, *26*(3), 487–499. https://doi.org/10.1016/S0005-7894(05)80096-6

Foa, E. B., & Rothbaum, B. O. (1989). Behavioural psychotherapy for post-traumatic stress disorder. *International Review of Psychiatry, 1*(3), 219–226. https://doi.org/10.3109/09540268909110412

Foa, E. B., & Rothbaum, B. O. (1998). *Treating the trauma of rape: Cognitive-behavior therapy for PTSD.* Guilford Press.

Foa, E. B., Rothbaum, B. O., Riggs, D. S., & Murdock, T. B. (1991). Treatment of post-traumatic stress disorder in rape victims: A comparison between cognitive-behavioral procedures and counseling. *Journal of Consulting and Clinical Psychology, 59*(5), 715–723. https://doi.org/10.1037/0022-006X.59.5.715

Foa, E. B., Stein, D. J., & McFarlane, A. C. (2006). Symptomatology and psychopathology of mental health problems after disaster. *Journal of Clinical Psychology, 67*(Suppl. 2), 15–25.

Foa, E., Steketee, G., & Rothbaum, B. O. (1989). Behavioral/cognitive conceptualizations of post-traumatic stress disorder. *Behavior Therapy, 20*(2), 155–176. Advance online publication. https://doi.org/10.1016/S0005-7894(89)80067-X

Foa, E. B., Yusko, D. A., McLean, C. P., Suvak, M. K., Bux, D. A., Jr., Oslin, D., O'Brien, C. P., Imms, P., Riggs, D. S., & Volpicelli, J. (2013). Concurrent naltrexone and prolonged exposure therapy for patients with comorbid alcohol dependence and PTSD: A randomized clinical trial. *Journal of the American Medical Association, 310*(5), 488–495. https://doi.org/10.1001/jama.2013.8268

Foa, E. B., Zandberg, L. J., McLean, C. P., Rosenfield, D., Fitzgerald, H., Tuerk, P. W., Wangelin, B. C., Young-McCaughan, S., & Peterson, A. L. (2019). The efficacy of 90-minute versus 60-minute sessions of prolonged exposure for posttraumatic stress disorder: Design of a randomized controlled trial in active duty military personnel. *Psychological Trauma: Theory, Research, Practice, and Policy, 11*(3), 307–313. https://doi.org/10.1037/tra0000351

Fonzo, G. A., Goodkind, M. S., Oathes, D. J., Zaiko, Y. V., Harvey, M., Peng, K. K., Weiss, M. E., Thompson, A. L., Zack, S. E., Lindley, S. E., Arnow, B. A., Jo, B., Gross, J. J., Rothbaum, B. O., & Etkin, A. (2017). PTSD psychotherapy outcome predicted by brain activation during emotional reactivity and regulation. *American Journal of Psychiatry, 174*(12), 1163–1174. https://doi.org/10.1176/appi.ajp.2017.16091072

Franke, L. M., Walker, W. C., Hoke, K. W., & Wares, J. R. (2016). Distinction in EEG slow oscillations between chronic mild traumatic brain injury and PTSD. *International Journal of Psychophysiology, 106*, 21–29. https://doi.org/10.1016/j.ijpsycho.2016.05.010

Freeman, D., Garety, P. A., Kuipers, E., Fowler, D., Bebbington, P. E., & Dunn, G. (2007). Acting on persecutory delusions: The importance of safety seeking. *Behaviour Research and Therapy, 45*(1), 89–99. https://doi.org/10.1016/j.brat.2006.01.014

Fryml, L. D., Pelic, C. G., Acierno, R., Tuerk, P., Yoder, M., Borckardt, J. J., Juneja, N., Shmidt, M., Beaver, K., George, M. S. (2019). Exposure therapy and simultaneous repetitive transcranial magnetic stimulation: A controlled pilot trial for the treatment of posttraumatic stress disorder. *Journal of ECT, 35*(1), 53–60.

Galatzer-Levy, I. R., & Bryant, R. A. (2013). 636,120 Ways to have posttraumatic stress disorder. *Perspectives on Psychological Science, 8*(6), 651–662. https://doi.org/10.1177/1745691613504115

Galatzer-Levy, I. R., Karstoft, K. I., Statnikov, A., & Shalev, A. Y. (2014). Quantitative forecasting of PTSD from early trauma responses: A machine learning application.

Journal of Psychiatric Research, *59*, 68–76. https://doi.org/10.1016/j.jpsychires.2014.08.017

Galatzer-Levy, I. R., Steenkamp, M. M., Brown, A. D., Qian, M., Inslicht, S., Henn-Haase, C., Otte, C., Yehuda, R., Neylan, T. C., & Marmar, C. R. (2014). Cortisol response to an experimental stress paradigm prospectively predicts long-term distress and resilience trajectories in response to active police service. *Journal of Psychiatric Research*, *56*, 36–42. https://doi.org/10.1016/j.jpsychires.2014.04.020

Garcia, N. M., Walker, R. S., & Zoellner, L. A. (2018). Estrogen, progesterone, and the menstrual cycle: A systematic review of fear learning, intrusive memories, and PTSD. *Clinical Psychology Review*, *66*, 80–96. https://doi.org/10.1016/j.cpr.2018.06.005

Garfinkel, S. N., Abelson, J. L., King, A. P., Sripada, R. K., Wang, X., Gaines, L. M., & Liberzon, I. (2014). Impaired contextual modulation of memories in PTSD: An fMRI and psychophysiological study of extinction retention and fear renewal. *Journal of Neuroscience*, *34*(40), 13435–13443. https://doi.org/10.1523/JNEUROSCI.4287-13.2014

Gerardi, M., Rothbaum, B. O., Astin, M. C., & Kelley, M. (2010). Cortisol response following exposure treatment for PTSD in rape victims. *Journal of Aggression, Maltreatment & Trauma*, *19*(4), 349–356. https://doi.org/10.1080/10926771003781297

Gomez, P., Ratcliff, R., & Perea, M. (2007). A model of the go/no-go task. *Journal of Experimental Psychology: General*, *136*(3), 389–413. https://doi.org/10.1037/0096-3445.136.3.389

Gonzalez-Lima, F., & Bruchey, A. K. (2004). Extinction memory improvement by the metabolic enhancer methylene blue. *Learning & Memory*, *11*(5), 633–640. https://doi.org/10.1101/lm.82404

Goodson, J. T., & Haeffel, G. J. (2018). Preventative and restorative safety behaviors: Effects on exposure treatment outcomes and risk for future anxious symptoms. *Journal of Clinical Psychology*, *74*, 1657–1672. Advance online publication. https://doi.org/10.1002/jclp.22635

Graham, B. M., & Milad, M. R. (2011). The study of fear extinction: Implications for anxiety disorders. *American Journal of Psychiatry*, *168*(12), 1255–1265. https://doi.org/10.1176/appi.ajp.2011.11040557

Gray, M. J., & Lombardo, T. W. (2001). Complexity of trauma narratives as an index of fragmented memory in PTSD: A critical analysis. *Applied Cognitive Psychology*, *15*(7), S171–S186. https://doi.org/10.1002/acp.840

Grayson, J. B., Foa, E. B., & Steketee, G. (1982). Habituation during exposure treatment: Distraction vs. attention-focusing. *Behaviour Research and Therapy*, *20*(4), 323–328. https://doi.org/10.1016/0005-7967(82)90091-2

Gressier, F., Calati, R., Balestri, M., Marsano, A., Alberti, S., Antypa, N., & Serretti, A. (2013). The 5-HTTLPR polymorphism and posttraumatic stress disorder: A meta-analysis. *Journal of Traumatic Stress*, *26*(6), 645–653. https://doi.org/10.1002/jts.21855

Gros, D. F., Yoder, M., Tuerk, P. W., Lozano, B. E., & Acierno, R. (2011). Exposure therapy for PTSD delivered to veterans via telehealth: Predictors of treatment completion and outcome and comparison to treatment delivered in person. *Behavior Therapy*, *42*(2), 276–283. https://doi.org/10.1016/j.beth.2010.07.005

Gunduz-Cinar, O., MacPherson, K. P., Cinar, R., Gamble-George, J., Sugden, K., Williams, B., Godlewski, G., Ramikie, T. S., Gorka, A. X., Alapafuja, S. O., Nikas, S. P.,

Makriyannis, A., Poulton, R., Patel, S., Hariri, A. R., Caspi, A., Moffitt, T. E., Kunos, G., & Holmes, A. (2013). Convergent translational evidence of a role for anandamide in amygdala-mediated fear extinction, threat processing and stress-reactivity. *Molecular Psychiatry, 18*(7), 813–823. https://doi.org/10.1038/mp.2012.72

Gutner, C. A., Suvak, M. K., Sloan, D. M., & Resick, P. A. (2016). Does timing matter? Examining the impact of session timing on outcome. *Journal of Consulting and Clinical Psychology, 84*(12), 1108–1115. https://doi.org/10.1037/ccp0000120

Hagenaars, M. A., van Minnen, A., & Hoogduin, K. A. L. (2010). The impact of dissociation and depression on the efficacy of prolonged exposure treatment for PTSD. *Behaviour Research and Therapy, 48*(1), 1927.

Halligan, S. L., Michael, T., Clark, D. M., & Ehlers, A. (2003). Posttraumatic stress disorder following assault: The role of cognitive processing, trauma memory, and appraisals. *Journal of Consulting and Clinical Psychology, 71*(3), 419–431. https://doi.org/10.1037/0022-006X.71.3.419

Hammoud, M. Z., Peters, C., Hatfield, J. R. B., Gorka, S. M., Phan, K. L., Milad, M. R., & Rabinak, C. A. (2019). Influence of Δ9-tetrahydrocannabinol on long-term neural correlates of threat extinction memory retention in humans. *Neuropsychopharmacology, 44*(10), 1769–1777. https://doi.org/10.1038/s41386-019-0416-6

Harned, M. S., Korslund, K. E., Foa, E. B., & Linehan, M. M. (2012). Treating PTSD in suicidal and self-injuring women with borderline personality disorder: Development and preliminary evaluation of a Dialectical Behavior Therapy Prolonged Exposure Protocol. *Behavior Research and Therapy, 50*(6), 381–386. https://doi.org/10.1016/j.brat.2012.02.011

Harned, M. S., Korslund, K. E., & Linehan, M. M. (2014). A pilot randomized controlled trial of dialectical behavior therapy with and without the dialectical behavior therapy prolonged exposure protocol for suicidal and self-injuring women with borderline personality disorder and PTSD. *Behaviour Research and Therapy, 55*, 7–17. https://doi.org/10.1016/j.brat.2014.01.008

Harned, M. S., Ruork, A. K., Liu, J., & Tkachuck, M. A. (2015). Emotional activation and habituation during imaginal exposure for PTSD among women with borderline personality disorder. *Journal of Traumatic Stress, 28*(3), 253–257.

Hauenstein, E. J., Petterson, S., Merwin, E., Rovnyak, V., Heise, B., & Wagner, D. (2006). Rurality, gender, and mental health treatment. *Family & Community Health, 29*(3), 169–185. https://doi.org/10.1097/00003727-200607000-00004

Hauer, D., Kaufmann, I., Strewe, C., Briegel, I., Campolongo, P., & Schelling, G. (2014). The role of glucocorticoids, catecholamines and endocannabinoids in the development of traumatic memories and posttraumatic stress symptoms in survivors of critical illness. *Neurobiology of Learning and Memory, 112*, 68–74. https://doi.org/10.1016/j.nlm.2013.10.003

Hayes, J. P., Hayes, S. M., & Mikedis, A. M. (2012). Quantitative meta-analysis of neural activity in posttraumatic stress disorder. *Biology of Mood & Anxiety Disorders, 2*, 9. https://doi.org/10.1186/2045-5380-2-9

Hembree, E. A., Foa, E. B., Dorfan, N. M., Street, G. P., Kowalski, J., & Tu, X. (2003). Do patients drop out prematurely from exposure therapy for PTSD? *Journal of Traumatic Stress, 16*(6), 555–562. https://doi.org/10.1023/B:JOTS.0000004078.93012.7d

Hendriks, G.-J., De Kleine, R., & Van Minnen, A. (2015). Optimizing the efficacy of exposure in PTSD treatment. *European Journal of Psychotraumatology, 6*(1). https://doi.org/10.3402/ejpt.v6.27628

Hendriks, L., de Kleine, R., Broekman, T., Hendriks, G., & van Minnen, A. (2018). Intensive prolonged exposure therapy for chronic PTSD patients following multiple trauma and multiple treatment attempts. *European Journal of Pharmacology, 9*(1). https://doi.org/10.1080/20008198.2018.1425574

Hepner, K. A., Farris, C., Farmer, C. M., Iyiewuare, P. O., Tanielian, T., Wilks, A., Robbins, M., Paddock, S. M., & Pincus, H. A. (2018). Delivering clinical practice guideline-concordant care for PTSD and major depression in military treatment facilities. *Rand Health Quarterly, 7*(3), 3.

Hermans, D., Dirikx, T., Vansteenwegen, D., Baeyens, F., Van den Bergh, O., & Eelen, P. (2005). Reinstatement of fear responses in human aversive conditioning. *Behaviour Research and Therapy, 43*(4), 533–551. https://doi.org/10.1016/j.brat.2004.03.013

Hernandez-Tejada, M. A., Acierno, R., & Sanchez-Carracedo, D. (2017). Addressing dropout from prolonged exposure: Feasibility of involving peers during exposure trials. *Military Psychology, 29*(2), 157–163.

Hernandez-Tejada, M. A., Acierno, R., & Sánchez-Carracedo, D. (2020). Re-engaging dropouts of prolonged exposure for ptsd delivered via home-based telemedicine or in person: Satisfaction with veteran-to-veteran support. *Journal of Behavioral Health Services and Research*, 1–12.

Hernandez-Tejada, M. A., Muzzy, W., Price, M., Hamski, S., Hart, S., Foa, E., & Acierno, R. (2020). Peer support during in vivo exposure homework to reverse attrition from prolonged exposure therapy for posttraumatic stress disorder (PTSD): Description of a randomized controlled trial. *Trials, 21*, 1–11.

Hinrichs, R., Michopoulos, V., Winters, S., Rothbaum, A. O., Rothbaum, B. O., Ressler, K. J., & Jovanovic, T. (2017). Mobile assessment of heightened skin conductance in posttraumatic stress disorder. *Depression and Anxiety, 34*(6), 502–507. https://doi.org/10.1002/da.22610

Hobfoll, S. E., Blais, R. K., Stevens, N. R., Walt, L., & Gengler, R. (2016). Vets Prevail online intervention reduces PTSD and depression in veterans with mild-to-moderate symptoms. *Journal of Consulting and Clinical Psychology, 84*(1), 31–42. https://doi.org/10.1037/ccp0000041

Hollifield, M. (2011). Acupuncture for posttraumatic stress disorder: Conceptual, clinical, and biological data support further research. *CNS Neuroscience & Therapeutics, 17*(6), 769–779. https://doi.org/10.1111/j.1755-5949.2011.00241.x

Hood, H. K., Antony, M. M., Koerner, N., & Monson, C. M. (2010). Effects of safety behaviors on fear reduction during exposure. *Behaviour Research and Therapy, 48*(12), 1161–1169. https://doi.org/10.1016/j.brat.2010.08.006

Horowitz, M. J. (1986). *Stress response syndromes* (2nd ed.). Aronson.

Hughes, K. C., & Shin, L. M. (2011). Functional neuroimaging studies of post-traumatic stress disorder. *Expert Review of Neurotherapeutics, 11*(2), 275–285. https://doi.org/10.1586/ern.10.198

Hussain, M., Al-Haiqi, A., Zaidan, A. A., Zaidan, B. B., Kiah, M. L. M., Anuar, N. B., & Abdulnabi, M. (2015). The landscape of research on smartphone medical apps: Coherent taxonomy, motivations, open challenges and recommendations. *Computer Methods and Programs in Biomedicine, 122*(3), 393–408. https://doi.org/10.1016/j.cmpb.2015.08.015

Im, J. J., Kim, B., Hwang, J., Kim, J. E., Kim, J. Y., Rhie, S. J., Namgung, E., Kang, I., Moon, S., Lyoo, I. K., Park, C. H., & Yoon, S. (2017). Diagnostic potential of multimodal neuroimaging in posttraumatic stress disorder. *PLOS ONE, 12*(5), e0177847. https://doi.org/10.1371/journal.pone.0177847

Imel, Z. E., Laska, K., Jakupcak, M., & Simpson, T. L. (2013). Meta-analysis of dropout in treatments for posttraumatic stress disorder. *Journal of Consulting and Clinical Psychology, 81*(3), 394–404. https://doi.org/10.1037/a0031474

International Society for Traumatic Stress Studies (ISTSS). (2018). *ISTSS PTSD prevention and treatment guidelines: Methodology and recommendations.* https://www.istss.org/getattachment/TreatingTrauma/New-ISTSS-Prevention-and-Treatment-Guidelines/ISTSS_ PreventionTreatmentGuidelines_FNL-March-19–2019.pdf.aspx

Isserles, M., Shalev, A. Y., Roth, Y., Peri, T., Kutz, I., Zlotnick, E., & Zangen, A. (2013). Effectiveness of deep transcranial magnetic stimulation combined with a brief exposure procedure in post-traumatic stress disorder—A pilot study. *Brain Stimulation, 6*(3), 377–383. https://doi.org/10.1016/j.brs.2012.07.008

Ivarsson, D., Blom, M., Hesser, H., Carlbring, P., Enderby, P., Nordberg, R., & Andersson, G. (2014). Guided internet-delivered cognitive behavior therapy for post-traumatic stress disorder: A randomized controlled trial. *Internet Interventions: The Application of Information Technology in Mental and Behavioural Health, 1*(1), 33–40. https://doi.org/10.1016/j.invent.2014.03.002

Jaeger, J., Lindblom, K. M., Parker-Guilbert, K., & Zoellner, L. A. (2014). Trauma narratives: It's what you say, not how you say it. *Psychological Trauma: Theory, Research, Practice, and Policy, 6*(5), 473–481. https://doi.org/10.1037/a0035239

Jang, K. L., Taylor, S., Stein, M. B., & Yamagata, S. (2007). Trauma exposure and stress response: Exploration of mechanisms of cause and effect. *Twin Research and Human Genetics, 10*(4), 564–572. https://doi.org/10.1375/twin.10.4.564

Janoff-Bulman, R. (1989). Assumptive worlds and the stress of traumatic events: Applications of the schema construct. *Social Cognition, 7*(2), 113–136. https://doi.org/10.1521/soco.1989.7.2.113

Jayakody, K., Gunadasa, S., & Hosker, C. (2014). Exercise for anxiety disorders: Systematic review. *British Journal of Sports Medicine, 48*(3), 187–196.

Jaycox, L. H., & Foa, E. B. (1996). Obstacles in implementing exposure therapy for PTSD: Case discussions and practical solutions. *Clinical Psychology & Psychotherapy: An International Journal of Theory and Practice, 3*(3), 176–184.

Jaycox, L. H., Foa, E. B., & Morral, A. R. (1998). Influence of emotional engagement and habituation on exposure therapy for PTSD. *Journal of Consulting and Clinical Psychology, 66*(1), 185–192. https://doi.org/10.1037/0022-006X.66.1.185

Johansen, P. O., & Krebs, T. S. (2009). How could MDMA (ecstasy) help anxiety disorders? A neurobiological rationale. *Journal of Psychopharmacology, 23*(4), 389–391. https://doi.org/10.1177/0269881109102787

Jones, C., Harvey, A. G., & Brewin, C. R. (2007). The organisation and content of trauma memories in survivors of road traffic accidents. *Behaviour Research and Therapy, 45*(1), 151–162. https://doi.org/10.1016/j.brat.2006.02.004

Joshi, S. A., Duval, E. R., Sheynin, J., King, A. P., Phan, K. L., Martis, B., Porter, K., Liberzon, I., Rauch, S. A. M. (2020). Neural correlates of emotional reactivity and regulation associated with treatment response in a randomized clinical trial for posttraumatic stress disorder. *Psychiatry Research: Neuroimaging,* 111062. https://doi.org/10.1016/j.pscychresns.2020.111062

Jovanovic, T., & Norrholm, S. D. (2016). Human psychophysiology and PTSD. In I. Liberzon & K. J. Ressler (Eds.), *Neurobiology of PTSD: From brain to mind* (pp. 292–316). Oxford University Press.

Jovanovic, T., Norrholm, S. D., Blanding, N. Q., Davis, M., Duncan, E., Bradley, B., & Ressler, K. J. (2010). Impaired fear inhibition is a biomarker of PTSD but not depression. *Depression and Anxiety, 27*(3), 244–251. https://doi.org/10.1002/da.20663

Jovanovic, T., Norrholm, S. D., Fennell, J. E., Keyes, M., Fiallos, A. M., Myers, K. M., Davis, M., & Duncan, E. J. (2009). Posttraumatic stress disorder may be associated with impaired fear inhibition: Relation to symptom severity. *Psychiatry Research, 167*(1–2), 151–160. https://doi.org/10.1016/j.psychres.2007.12.014

Kaczkurkin, A. N., Burton, P. C., Chazin, S. M., Manbeck, A. B., Espensen-Sturges, T., Cooper, S. E., Sponheim, S. R., & Lissek, S. (2017). Neural substrates of overgeneralized conditioned fear in PTSD. *American Journal of Psychiatry, 174*(2), 125–134. https://doi.org/10.1176/appi.ajp.2016.15121549

Kamphuis, J. H., & Telch, M. J. (2000). Effects of distraction and guided threat reappraisal on fear reduction during exposure-based treatments for specific fears. *Behaviour Research and Therapy, 38*(12), 1163–1181. https://doi.org/10.1016/S0005-7967(99)00147-3

Keane, T. M., & Barlow, D. H. (2002). Posttraumatic stress disorder. In D. H. Barlow (Ed.), *Anxiety and its disorders* (pp. 418–453). Guilford Press.

Keane, T. M., Fairbank, J. A., Caddell, J. M., & Zimering, R. T. (1989). Implosive (flooding) therapy reduces symptoms of PTSD in Vietnam combat veterans. *Behavior Therapy, 20*(2), 245–260. https://doi.org/10.1016/S0005-7894(89)80072-3

Keane, T. M., Kolb, L. C., Kaloupek, D. G., Orr, S. P., Blanchard, E. B., Thomas, R. G., Hsieh, F. Y., & Lavori, P. W. (1998). Utility of psychophysiological measurement in the diagnosis of posttraumatic stress disorder: Results from a Department of Veterans Affairs Cooperative Study. *Journal of Consulting and Clinical Psychology, 66*(6), 914–923. https://doi.org/10.1037/0022-006X.66.6.914

Keane, T. M., Zimering, R. T., & Caddell, J. M. (1985). A behavioral formulation of posttraumatic stress disorder in Vietnam veterans. *Behavior Therapist, 8*(1), 9–12.

Keefe, J. R., Wiltsey Stirman, S., Cohen, Z. D., DeRubeis, R. J., Smith, B. N., & Resick, P. A. (2018). In rape trauma PTSD, patient characteristics indicate which trauma-focused treatment they are most likely to complete. *Depression and Anxiety, 35*(4), 330–338. https://doi.org/10.1002/da.22731

Kehle-Forbes, S. M., Meis, L. A., Spoont, M. R., & Polusny, M. A. (2016). Treatment initiation and dropout from prolonged exposure and cognitive processing therapy in a VA outpatient clinic. *Psychological Trauma: Theory, Research, Practice, and Policy, 8*(1), 107–114. https://doi.org/10.1037/tra0000065

Kehle-Forbes, S. M., Polusny, M. A., MacDonald, R., Murdoch, M., Meis, L. A., & Wilt, T. J. (2013). A systematic review of the efficacy of adding nonexposure components to exposure therapy for posttraumatic stress disorder. *Psychological Trauma: Theory, Research, Practice, and Policy, 5*(4), 317–322. https://doi.org/10.1037/a0030040

Khan, N. I., Burkhouse, K. L., Lieberman, L., Gorka, S. M., DiGangi, J. A., Schroth, C., & Phan, K. L. (2018). Individual differences in combat experiences and error-related brain activity in OEF/OIF/OND veterans. *International Journal of Psychophysiology, 129*, 52–57. https://doi.org/10.1016/j.ijpsycho.2018.04.011

Kilpatrick, D. G., Veronen, L. J., & Best, C. L. (1985). Factors predicting psychological distress among rape victims. In Figley, C. R. (Ed.), *Trauma and its wake* (pp. 113–141). Brunner/Mazel.

Kindt, M., Buck, N., Arntz, A., & Soeter, M. (2007). Perceptual and conceptual processing as predictors of treatment outcome in PTSD. *Journal of Behavior Therapy and Experimental Psychiatry, 38*(4), 491–506. https://doi.org/10.1016/j.jbtep.2007.10.002

King, A. P., Abelson, J. L., Britton, J. C., Phan, K. L., Taylor, S. F., & Liberzon, I. (2009). Medial prefrontal cortex and right insula activity predict plasma ACTH response to trauma recall. *NeuroImage, 47*(3), 872–880. https://doi.org/10.1016/j.neuroimage.2009.05.088

Kircanski, K., Mortazavi, A., Castriotta, N., Baker, A. S., Mystkowski, J. L., Yi, R., & Craske, M. G. (2012). Challenges to the traditional exposure paradigm: Variability in exposure therapy for contamination fears. *Journal of Behavior Therapy and Experimental Psychiatry, 43*(2), 745–751. https://doi.org/10.1016/j.jbtep.2011.10.010

Klengel, T., Mehta, D., Anacker, C., Rex-Haffner, M., Pruessner, J. C., Pariante, C. M., Pace, T. W., Mercer, K. B., Mayberg, H. S., Bradley, B., Nemeroff, C. B., Holsboer, F., Heim, C. M., Ressler, K. J., Rein, T., & Binder, E. B. (2013). Allele-specific FKBP5 DNA demethylation mediates gene-childhood trauma interactions. *Nature Neuroscience, 16*(1), 33–41. https://doi.org/10.1038/nn.3275

Klumpers, F., Denys, D., Kenemans, J. L., Grillon, C., van der Aart, J., & Baas, J. M. (2012). Testing the effects of Δ9-THC and D-cycloserine on extinction of conditioned fear in humans. *Journal of Psychopharmacology, 26*(4), 471–478. https://doi.org/10.1177/0269881111431624

Knaevelsrud, C., Brand, J., Lange, A., Ruwaard, J., & Wagner, B. (2015). Web-based psychotherapy for posttraumatic stress disorder in war-traumatized Arab patients: Randomized controlled trial. *Journal of Medical Internet Research, 17*(3), e71.

Knowles, K. A., Sripada, R. K., Defever, M., & Rauch, S. A. M. (2019). Comorbid mood and anxiety disorders and severity of posttraumatic stress disorder symptoms in treatment-seeking veterans. *Psychological Trauma: Theory, Research, Practice, and Policy, 11*(4), 451–458. https://doi.org/10.1037/tra0000383

Koenen, K. C., Ratanatharathorn, A., Ng, L., McLaughlin, K. A., Bromet, E. J., Stein, D. J., Karam, E. G., Meron Ruscio, A., Benjet, C., Scott, K., Atwoli, L., Petukhova, M., Lim, C. C. W., Aguilar-Gaxiola, S., Al-Hamzawi, A., Alonso, J., Bunting, B., Ciutan, M., de Girolamo, G., . . . Kessler, R. C. (2017). Posttraumatic stress disorder in the world mental health surveys. *Psychological Medicine, 47*(13), 2260–2274. https://doi.org/10.1017/S0033291717000708

Kozak, M. J., Foa, E. B., & Steketee, G. (1988). Process and outcome of exposure treatment with obsessive-compulsives: Psychophysiological indicators of emotional processing. *Behavior Therapy, 19*(2), 157–169. https://doi.org/10.1016/S0005-7894(88)80039-X

Kozel, F. A., Motes, M. A., Didehbani, N., DeLaRosa, B., Bass, C., Schraufnagel, Jones, P., Morgan, C. R., Spence, J. S., Kraut, M. A., & Hart, J. (2018). Repetitive TMS to augment cognitive processing therapy in combat veterans of recent conflicts with PTSD: A randomized clinical trial. *Journal of Affective Disorders, 229*, 506–514.

Kredlow, A. M., Pineles, S. L., Inslicht, S. S., Marin, M.-F., Milad, M. R., Otto, M. W., & Orr, S. P. (2017). Assessment of skin conductance in African American and non-African American participants in studies of conditioned fear. *Psychophysiology*, *54*(11), 1741–1754. https://doi.org/10.1111/psyp.12909

Krupnick, J. L., Green, B. L., Amdur, R., Alaoui, A., Belouali, A., Roberge, E., Cueva, D., Roberts, M., Melnikoff, E., & Dutton, M. A. (2017). An internet-based writing intervention for PTSD in veterans: A feasibility and pilot effectiveness trial. *Psychological Trauma: Theory, Research, Practice, and Policy*, *9*(4), 461–470. https://doi.org/10.1037/tra0000176

Kuhn, E., Crowley, J. J., Hoffman, J. E., Eftekhari, A., Ramsey, K. M., Owen, J. E., & Ruzek, J. I. (2015). Clinician characteristics and perceptions related to use of the PE (prolonged exposure) Coach mobile app. *Professional Psychology, Research and Practice*, *46*(6), 437–443. https://doi.org/10.1037/pro0000051

Kuhn, E., Kanuri, N., Hoffman, J. E., Garvert, D. W., Ruzek, J. I., & Taylor, C. B. (2017). A randomized controlled trial of a smartphone app for posttraumatic stress disorder symptoms. *Journal of Consulting and Clinical Psychology*, *85*(3), 267.

Kumpula, M. J., Pentel, K. Z., Foa, E. B., LeBlanc, N. J., Bui, E., McSweeney, L. B., & Rauch, S. A. (2017). Temporal sequencing of change in posttraumatic cognitions and PTSD symptom reduction during prolonged exposure therapy. *Behavior Therapy*, *48*(2), 156–165.

Kutas, M., & Federmeier, K. D. (2011). Thirty years and counting: Finding meaning in the N400 component of the event-related brain potential (ERP). *Annual Review of Psychology*, *62*, 621–647. https://doi.org/10.1146/annurev.psych.093008.131123

Lang, A. J. & Craske, M. G. (2000). Manipulations of exposure-based therapy to reduce return of fear: A replication. *Behaviour Research and Therapy*, *38*(1), 1–12. https://doi.org/10.1016/S0005-7967(99)00031-5

Lang, P. J. (1977). Imagery in therapy: An information processing analysis of fear. *Behavior Therapy*, *8*(5), 862–886. https://doi.org/10.1016/S0005-7894(77)80157-3

Lang, P. J. (1979). Presidential address, 1978: A bio-informational theory of emotional imagery. *Psychophysiology*, *16*, 495–512. https://doi.org/10.1111/j.1469-8986.1979.tb01511.x

Lang, P. J., Melamed, B. G., & Hart, J. (1970). A psychophysiological analysis of fear modification using an automated desensitization procedure. *Journal of Abnormal Psychology*, *76*(2), 220–234. https://doi.org/10.1037/h0029875

Langkaas, T. F., Hoffart, A., Øktedalen, T., Ulvenes, P. G., Hembree, E. A., & Smucker, M. (2017). Exposure and non-fear emotions: A randomized controlled study of exposure-based and rescripting-based imagery in PTSD treatment. *Behaviour Research and Therapy*, *97*, 33–42. https://doi.org/10.1016/j.brat.2017.06.007

Lanius, R. A., Frewen, P. A., Tursich, M., Jetly, R., & McKinnon, M. C. (2015). Restoring large-scale brain networks in PTSD and related disorders: A proposal for neuroscientifically-informed treatment interventions. *European Journal of Psychotraumatology*, *6*(1), 27313. https://doi.org/10.3402/ejpt.v6.27313

Lazarov, A., Zhu, X., Suarez-Jimenez, B., Rutherford, B. R., & Neria, Y. (2017). Resting-state functional connectivity of anterior and posterior hippocampus in posttraumatic stress disorder. *Journal of Psychiatric Research*, *94*, 15–22. https://doi.org/10.1016/j.jpsychires.2017.06.003

Lee, C., Gavriel, H., Drummond, P., Richards, J., & Greenwald, R. (2002). Treatment of PTSD: Stress inoculation training with prolonged exposure compared to EMDR. *Journal of Clinical Psychology, 58*(9), 1071–1089. https://doi.org/10.1002/jclp.10039

Lee, S.-H., Yoon, S., Kim, J.-I., Jin, S.-H., & Chung, C. K. (2014). Functional connectivity of resting state EEG and symptom severity in patients with post-traumatic stress disorder. *Progress in Neuro-Psychopharmacology and Biological Psychiatry, 51*, 51–57. https://doi.org/10.1016/j.pnpbp.2014.01.008

Lewis, C. E., Farewell, D., Groves, V., Kitchiner, N. J., Roberts, N. P., Vick, T., & Bisson, J. I. (2017). Internet-based guided self-help for posttraumatic stress disorder: Randomized controlled trial. *Depression and Anxiety, 34*(6), 555–565. https://doi.org/10.1002/da.22645

Lewis, C. E., Roberts, N. P., Simon, N., Bethell, A., & Bisson, J. I. (2019). Internet-delivered cognitive behavioural therapy for post-traumatic stress disorder (PTSD): Systematic review and meta-analysis. *Acta Psychiatrica Scandinavica, 140*(6), 508–521.

Liberzon, I., & Abelson, J. L. (2016). Context processing and the neurobiology of post-traumatic stress disorder. *Neuron, 92*(1), 14–30. https://doi.org/10.1016/j.neuron.2016.09.039

Liberzon, I., King, A. P., Ressler, K. J., Almli, L. M., Zhang, P., Ma, S. T., Cohen, G. H., Tamburrino, M. B., Calabrese, J. R., & Galea, S. (2014). Interaction of the ADRB2 gene polymorphism with childhood trauma in predicting adult symptoms of post-traumatic stress disorder. *JAMA Psychiatry, 71*(10), 1174–1182. https://doi.org/10.1001/jamapsychiatry.2014.999

Linardon, J., Cuijpers, P., Carlbring, P., Messer, M., & Fuller-Tyszkiewicz, M. (2019). The efficacy of app-supported smartphone interventions for mental health problems: A meta-analysis of randomized controlled trials. *World Psychiatry, 18*(3), 325–336. https://doi.org/10.1002/wps.20673

Linehan, M. M., Comtois, K. A., Murray, A. M., Brown, M. Z., Gallop, R. J., Heard, H. L., Korslund, K. E., Tutek, D. A., Reynolds, S. K., & Lindenboim, N. (2006). Two-year randomized controlled trial and follow-up of dialectical behavior therapy vs therapy by experts for suicidal behaviors and borderline personality disorder. *Archives of General Psychiatry, 63*(7), 757–766. https://doi.org/10.1001/archpsyc.63.7.757

Linnman, C., Zeffiro, T. A., Pitman, R. K., & Milad, M. R. (2011). An fMRI study of unconditioned responses in post-traumatic stress disorder. *Biology of Mood & Anxiety Disorders, 1*(1), 8. https://doi.org/10.1186/2045-5380-1-8

Liriano, F., Hatten, C., & Schwartz, T. L. (2019). Ketamine as treatment for post-traumatic stress disorder: A review. *Drugs in Context, 8*, 212305. https://doi.org/10.7573/dic.212305

Lissek, S., Biggs, A. L., Rabin, S. J., Cornwell, B. R., Alvarez, R. P., Pine, D. S., & Grillon, C. (2008). Generalization of conditioned fear-potentiated startle in humans: Experimental validation and clinical relevance. *Behaviour Research and Therapy, 46*(5), 678–687. https://doi.org/10.1016/j.brat.2008.02.005

Lissek, S., Rabin, S., Heller, R. E., Lukenbaugh, D., Geraci, M., Pine, D. S., & Grillon, C. (2010). Overgeneralization of conditioned fear as a pathogenic marker of panic disorder. *American Journal of Psychiatry, 167*(1), 47–55. https://doi.org/10.1176/appi.ajp.2009.09030410

Lissek, S., & van Meurs, B. (2015). Learning models of PTSD: Theoretical accounts and psychobiological evidence. *International Journal of Psychophysiology, 98*(3, Pt. 2), 594–605. https://doi.org/10.1016/j.ijpsycho.2014.11.006

Litz, B. T., Engel, C. C., Bryant, R. A., & Papa, A. (2007). A randomized, controlled proof-of-concept trial of an internet-based, therapist-assisted self-management treatment for posttraumatic stress disorder. *American Journal of Psychiatry, 164*, 1676–1683. https://doi.org/10.1176/appi.ajp.2007.06122057

Litz, B. T., Salters-Pedneault, K., Steenkamp, M. M., Hermos, J. A., Bryant, R. A., Otto, M. W., & Hofmann, S. G. (2012). A randomized placebo-controlled trial of D-cycloserine and exposure therapy for posttraumatic stress disorder. *Journal of Psychiatric Research, 46*(9), 1184–1190. https://doi.org/10.1016/j.jpsychires.2012.05.006

Liu, P. Z., & Nusslock, R. (2018). Exercise-mediated neurogenesis in the hippocampus via BDNF. *Frontiers in Neuroscience, 12*(52), 52. Advance online publication. https://doi.org/10.3389/fnins.2018.00052

Lobo, I., Portugal, L. C., Figueira, I., Volchan, E., David, I., Garcia Pereira, M., & de Oliveira, L. (2015). EEG correlates of the severity of posttraumatic stress symptoms: A systematic review of the dimensional PTSD literature. *Journal of Affective Disorders, 183*, 210–220. https://doi.org/10.1016/j.jad.2015.05.015

Lonergan, M. H., Olivera-Figueroa, L. A., Pitman, R. K., & Brunet, A. (2012). Propranolol's effects on the consolidation and reconsolidation of long-term emotional memory in healthy participants: A meta-analysis. *Journal of Psychiatry & Neuroscience, 38*(4), 222–231.

Loucks, L., Yasinski, C., Norrholm, S. D., Maples-Keller, J., Post, L., Zwiebach, L., Fiorillo, D., Goodlin, M., Jovanovic, T., Rizzo, A. A., & Rothbaum, B. O. (2019). You can do that?!: Feasibility of virtual reality exposure therapy in the treatment of PTSD due to military sexual trauma. *Journal of Anxiety Disorders, 61*, 55–63. https://doi.org/10.1016/j.janxdis.2018.06.004

MacLeod, C., Mathews, A., & Tata, P. (1986). Attentional bias in emotional disorders. *Journal of Abnormal Psychology, 95*(1), 15–20. https://doi.org/10.1037/0021-843X.95.1.15

Maples-Keller, J. L., Jovanovic, T., Dunlop, B. W., Rauch, S., Yasinski, C., Michopoulos, V., Coghlan, C., Norrholm, S., Rizzo, A. S., Ressler, K., & Rothbaum, B. O. (2019). When translational neuroscience fails in the clinic: Dexamethasone prior to virtual reality exposure therapy increases drop-out rates. *Journal of Anxiety Disorders, 61*, 89–97. https://doi.org/10.1016/j.janxdis.2018.10.006

Maples-Keller, J. L., Rauch, S. A. M., Jovanovic, T., Yasinski, C. W., Goodnight, J. M., Sherrill, A., Black, K., Michopoulos, V., Dunlop, B. W., Rothbaum, B. O., & Norrholm, S. D. (2019). Changes in trauma-potentiated startle, skin conductance, and heart rate within prolonged exposure therapy for PTSD in high and low treatment responders. *Journal of Anxiety Disorders, 68*, 102147. https://doi.org/10.1016/j.janxdis.2019.102147

Markowitz, J. C., Neria, Y., Lovell, K., Van Meter, P. E., & Petkova, E. (2017). History of sexual trauma moderates psychotherapy outcome for posttraumatic stress disorder. *Depression and Anxiety, 34*(8), 692–700. https://doi.org/10.1002/da.22619

Markowitz, J. C., Petkova, E., Neria, Y., Van Meter, P. E., Zhao, Y., Hembree, E., Lovell, K., Biyanova, T., & Marshall, R. D. (2015). Is exposure necessary? A randomized clinical trial of interpersonal psychotherapy for PTSD. *American Journal of Psychiatry, 172*(5), 430–440.

Marks, I., Lovell, K., Noshirvani, H., Livanou, M., & Thrasher, S. (1998). Treatment of posttraumatic stress disorder by exposure and/or cognitive restructuring: A controlled study. *Archives of General Psychiatry, 55*(4), 317–325. https://doi.org/10.1001/archpsyc.55.4.317

Marsicano, G., Wotjak, C. T., Azad, S. C., Bisogno, T., Rammes, G., Cascio, M. G., Hermann, H., Tang, J., Hofmann, C., Zieglgänsberger, W., Di Marzo, V., & Lutz, B. (2002). The endogenous cannabinoid system controls extinction of aversive memories. *Nature, 418*, 530–534. https://doi.org/10.1038/nature00839

Mason, J. W., Giller, E. L., Kosten, T. R., Ostroff, R. B., & Podd, L. (1986). Urinary free-cortisol levels in posttraumatic stress disorder patients. *Journal of Nervous and Mental Disease, 174*(3), 145–149. https://doi.org/10.1097/00005053-198603000-00003

Mason, J. W., Wang, S., Yehuda, R., Lubin, H., Johnson, D., Bremner, J. D., Charney, D., & Southwick, S. (2002). Marked lability in urinary cortisol levels in subgroups of combat veterans with posttraumatic stress disorder during an intensive exposure treatment program. *Psychosomatic Medicine, 64*(2), 238–246. https://doi.org/10.1097/00006842-200203000-00006

Mataix-Cols, D., Fernández de la Cruz, L., Monzani, B., Rosenfield, D., Andersson, E., Pérez-Vigil, A., Frumento, P., de Kleine, R. A., Difede, J., Dunlop, B. W., Farrell, L. J., Geller, D., Gerardi, M., Guastella, A. J., Hofmann, S. G., Hendriks, G. J., Kushner, M. G., Lee, F. S., Lenze, E. J., . . . the DCS Anxiety Consortium. (2017). D-cycloserine augmentation of exposure-based cognitive behavior therapy for anxiety, obsessive-compulsive, and posttraumatic stress disorders: A systematic review and meta-analysis of individual participant data. *JAMA Psychiatry, 74*(5), 501–510. https://doi.org/10.1001/jamapsychiatry.2016.3955

Matthews, A. R., He, O. H., Buhusi, M., & Buhusi, C. V. (2012). Dissociation of the role of the prelimbic cortex in interval timing and resource allocation: Beneficial effect of norepinephrine and dopamine reuptake inhibitor nomifensine on anxiety-inducing distraction. *Frontiers in Integrative Neuroscience, 6*, 111. https://doi.org/10.3389/fnint.2012.00111

McCann, I. L., & Pearlman, L. A. (1990). *Psychological trauma and the adult survivor: Theory, therapy, and transformation.* Brunner/Mazel.

McCann, I. L., Sakheim, D. K., & Abrahamson, D. J. (1988). Trauma and victimization. *Counseling Psychologist, 16*(4), 531–594. https://doi.org/10.1177/0011000088164002

McClendon, J., Dean, K. E., & Galovski, T. (2020). Addressing diversity in PTSD treatment: Disparities in treatment engagement and outcome among patients of color. *Current Treatment Options in Psychiatry, 7*, 275–290. Advance online publication. https://doi.org/10.1007/s40501-020-00212-0

McDonagh, A., Friedman, M., McHugo, G., Ford, J., Sengupta, A., Mueser, K., Demment, C. C., Fournier, D., Schnurr, P. P., & Descamps, M. (2005). Randomized trial of cognitive-behavioral therapy for chronic posttraumatic stress disorder in adult female survivors of childhood sexual abuse. *Journal of Consulting and Clinical Psychology, 73*(3), 515–524. https://doi.org/10.1037/0022-006X.73.3.515

McGhee, L. L., Maani, C. V., Garza, T. H., Gaylord, K. M., & Black, I. H. (2008). The correlation between ketamine and posttraumatic stress disorder in burned service members. *Journal of Trauma, 64*(Suppl.), S195–S199. https://doi.org/10.1097/TA.0b013e318160ba1d

McLaughlin, T., Blum, K., Oscar-Berman, M., Febo, M., Agan, G., Fratantonio, J. L., Simpatico, T., & Gold, M. S. (2015). Putative dopamine agonist (KB220Z) attenuates lucid nightmares in PTSD patients: Role of enhanced brain reward functional connectivity and homeostasis redeeming joy. *Journal of Behavioral Addictions, 4*(2), 106–115. https://doi.org/10.1556/2006.4.2015.008

McLean, C., P., Foa, E. B., Dondanville, K. A., Haddock, C. K., Miller, M. L., Rauch, S. A. M., Yarvis, J. S., Wright, E. C., Hall-Clark, B. N., Fina, B. A., Litz, B. T., Mintz, J., Young-McCaughan, S., & Peterson, A. L. (2020). The efficacy of web-prolonged exposure among military personnel and veterans with PTSD. *Psychological Trauma: Theory, Research, Practice, and Policy.* Advance online publication. https://doi.org/10.1037/tra0000978

McLean, C. P., Su, Y. J., & Foa, E. B. (2015). Mechanisms of symptom reduction in a combined treatment for comorbid posttraumatic stress disorder and alcohol dependence. *Journal of Consulting and Clinical Psychology, 83*(3), 655–661. https://doi.org/10.1037/ccp0000024

McLean, C. P., Yeh, R., Rosenfield, D., & Foa, E. B. (2015). Changes in negative cognitions mediate PTSD symptom reductions during client-centered therapy and prolonged exposure for adolescents. *Behaviour Research and Therapy, 68*, 64–69. https://doi.org/10.1016/j.brat.2015.03.008

McLean, C. P., Zang, Y., Gallagher, T., Suzuki, N., Yarvis, J. S., Litz, B. T., Mintz, J., Young-McCaughan, S., Peterson, A. L., Foa, E. B., & the STRONG STAR Consortium. (2019). Trauma-related cognitions and cognitive emotion regulation as mediators of PTSD change among treatment-seeking active-duty military personnel with PTSD. *Behavior Therapy, 50*(6), 1053–1062. https://doi.org/10.1016/j.beth.2019.03.006

McManus, F., Sacadura, C., & Clark, D. M. (2008). Why social anxiety persists: An experimental investigation of the role of safety behaviours as a maintaining factor. *Journal of Behavior Therapy and Experimental Psychiatry, 39*(2), 147–161. https://doi.org/10.1016/j.jbtep.2006.12.002

McRae-Clark, A. L., Baker, N. L., Maria, M. M., & Brady, K. T. (2013). Effect of oxytocin on craving and stress response in marijuana-dependent individuals: A pilot study. *Psychopharmacology, 228*(4), 623–631. https://doi.org/10.1007/s00213-013-3062-4

Mellon, S. H. (2007). Neurosteroid regulation of central nervous system development. *Pharmacology & Therapeutics, 116*(1), 107–124. https://doi.org/10.1016/j.pharmthera.2007.04.011

Mellon, S. H., Griffin, L. D., & Compagnone, N. A. (2001). Biosynthesis and action of neurosteroids. *Brain Research Reviews, 37*(1–3), 3–12. https://doi.org/10.1016/S0165-0173(01)00109-6

Meng, L., Jiang, J., Jin, C., Liu, J., Zhao, Y., Wang, W., Li, K., & Gong, Q. (2016). Trauma-specific grey matter alterations in PTSD. *Scientific Reports, 6*(1), 33748. https://doi.org/10.1038/srep33748

Merz, C. J., Hamacher-Dang, T. C., Stark, R., Wolf, O. T., & Hermann, A. (2018). Neural underpinnings of cortisol effects on fear extinction. *Neuropsychopharmacology, 43*(2), 384–392. https://doi.org/10.1038/npp.2017.227

Meuret, A. E., Seidel, A., Rosenfield, B., Hofmann, S. G., & Rosenfield, D. (2012). Does fear reactivity during exposure predict panic symptom reduction? *Journal of Consulting and Clinical Psychology, 80*(5), 773–785. https://doi.org/10.1037/a0028032

Michopoulos, V., Rothbaum, A. O., Jovanovic, T., Almli, L. M., Bradley, B., Rothbaum, B. O., Gillespie, C. F., & Ressler, K. J. (2015). Association of CRP genetic variation and CRP level with elevated PTSD symptoms and physiological responses in a civilian population with high levels of trauma. *American Journal of Psychiatry, 172*(4), 353–362. https://doi.org/10.1176/appi.ajp.2014.14020263

Milad, M. R., Pitman, R. K., Ellis, C. B., Gold, A. L., Shin, L. M., Lasko, N. B., Zeidan, M. A., Handwerger, K., Orr, S. P., & Rauch, S. L. (2009). Neurobiological basis of failure to recall extinction memory in posttraumatic stress disorder. *Biological Psychiatry, 66*(12), 1075–1082. https://doi.org/10.1016/j.biopsych.2009.06.026

Milad, M. R., Quirk, G. J., Pitman, R. K., Orr, S. P., Fischl, B., & Rauch, S. L. (2007). A role for the human dorsal anterior cingulate cortex in fear expression. *Biological Psychiatry, 62*(10), 1191–1194. https://doi.org/10.1016/j.biopsych.2007.04.032

Miller, J. K., McDougall, S., Thomas, S., & Wiener, J. (2017). The impact of the brain-derived neurotrophic factor gene on trauma and spatial processing. *Journal of Clinical Medicine, 6*(12), 108. https://doi.org/10.3390/jcm6120108

Miller, M., Davis, A., & McLean, C. (2020). Development and pilot testing of a trauma-focused cognitive-behavioral self-management mobile app for post-traumatic stress symptoms. *Journal of Technology in Behavioral Science.* https://doi.org/10.1007/s41347-020-00188-x

Mills, K. L., Teesson, M., Back, S. E., Brady, K. T., Baker, A. L., Hopwood, S., Sannibale, C., Barrett, E. L., Merz, S., Rosenfeld, J., & Ewer, P. L. (2012). Integrated exposure-based therapy for co-occurring posttraumatic stress disorder and substance dependence: A randomized controlled trial. *Journal of the American Medical Association, 308*(7), 690–699. https://doi.org/10.1001/jama.2012.9071

Milosevic, I., & Radomsky, A. S. (2008). Safety behaviour does not necessarily interfere with exposure therapy. *Behaviour Research and Therapy, 46*, 1111–1118. https://doi.org/10.1016/j.brat.2008.05.011

Miner, A., Kuhn, E., Hoffman, J. E., Owen, J. E., Ruzek, J. I., & Taylor, C. B. (2016). Feasibility, acceptability, and potential efficacy of the PTSD Coach app: A pilot randomized controlled trial with community trauma survivors. *Psychological Trauma: Theory, Research, Practice, and Policy, 8*(3), 384–392. https://doi.org/10.1037/tra0000092

Misaki, N., Higuchi, H., Yamagata, K., & Miki, N. (1992). Identification of glucocorticoid responsive elements (GREs) at far upstream of rat NPY gene. *Neurochemistry International, 21*(2), 185–189. https://doi.org/10.1016/0197–0186(92)90145-H

Mithoefer, M. C., Wagner, M. T., Mithoefer, A. T., Jerome, L., & Doblin, R. (2011). The safety and efficacy of +/–3,4-methylenedioxymethamphetamine-assisted psychotherapy in subjects with chronic, treatment-resistant posttraumatic stress disorder: The first randomized controlled pilot study. *Journal of Psychopharmacology, 25*(4), 439–452. https://doi.org/10.1177/0269881110378371

Mithoefer, M. C., Wagner, M. T., Mithoefer, A. T., Jerome, L., Martin, S. F., Yazar-Klosinski, B., Michel, Y., Brewerton, T. D., & Doblin, R. (2013). Durability of improvement in post-traumatic stress disorder symptoms and absence of harmful effects or drug dependency after 3,4-methylenedioxymethamphetamine-assisted psychotherapy: A prospective long-term follow-up study. *Journal of Psychopharmacology, 27*(1), 28–39. https://doi.org/10.1177/0269881112456611

Modarres, M. H., Opel, R. A., Weymann, K. B., & Lim, M. M. (2019). Strong correlation of novel sleep electroencephalography coherence markers with diagnosis and severity of posttraumatic stress disorder. *Scientific Reports*, *9*(1), 4247. https://doi. org/10.1038/s41598-018-38102-4

Morey, R. A., Dunsmoor, J. E., Haswell, C. C., Brown, V. M., Vora, A., Weiner, J., Stjepanovic, D., Wagner, H. R., III, LaBar, K. S., & the VA Mid-Atlantic MIRECC Workgroup. (2015). Fear learning circuitry is biased toward generalization of fear associations in posttraumatic stress disorder. *Translational Psychiatry*, *5*(12), e700. https://doi.org/10.1038/tp.2015.196

Morland, L. A., Greene, C. J., Rosen, C. S., Kuhn, E., Hoffman, J., & Sloan, D. M. (2017). Telehealth and eHealth interventions for posttraumatic stress disorder. *Current Opinion in Psychology*, *14*, 102–108. https://doi.org/10.1016/j.copsyc.2016. 12.003

Morland, L. A., Mackintosh, M. A., Glassman, L. H., Wells, S. Y., Thorp, S. R., Rauch, S. A., & Golshan, S. (2020). Home-based delivery of variable length prolonged exposure therapy: A comparison of clinical efficacy between service modalities. *Depression and Anxiety*, *37*(4), 346–355. https://doi.org/10.1002/da.22979.

Morrison, F. G., Miller, M. W., Logue, M. W., Assef, M., & Wolf, E. J. (2019). DNA methylation correlates of PTSD: Recent findings and technical challenges. *Progress in Neuro-Psychopharmacology & Biological Psychiatry*, *90*, 223–234. https://doi.org/ 10.1016/j.pnpbp.2018.11.011

Moulds, M. L., & Bryant, R. A. (2005). An investigation of retrieval inhibition in acute stress disorder. *Journal of Traumatic Stress*, *18*(3), 233–236. https://doi.org/10. 1002/jts.20022

Mowrer, O. H. (1960). *Learning theory and behavior*. John Wiley & Sons. https://doi. org/10.1037/10802-000

Mowrer, O. H., & Suter, J. W. (1950). *Further evidence for a two-factor theory of learning* [Unpublished manuscript].

Murray, J., Ehlers, A., & Mayou, R. A. (2002). Dissociation and post-traumatic stress disorder: Two prospective studies of road traffic accident survivors. *British Journal of Psychiatry*, *180*(4), 363–368. https://doi.org/10.1192/bjp.180.4.363

Myers, U. S., Keller, S. M., Grubaugh, A. L., & Tuerk, P. W. (2019). Prazosin use during prolonged exposure therapy with veterans: An examination of treatment effectiveness. *Military Behavioral Health*, *7*(1), 100–107.

Mystkowski, J. L., Craske, M. G., & Echiverri, A. M. (2002). Treatment context and return of fear in spider phobia. *Behavior Therapy*, *33*(3), 399–416. https://doi.org/ 10.1016/S0005–7894(02)80035–1

Mystkowski, J. L., Craske, M. G., Echiverri, A. M. L., & Labus, J. S. (2006). Mental reinstatement of context and return of fear in spider-fearful participants. *Behavior Therapy*, *37*(1), 49–60. https://doi.org/10.1016/j.beth.2005.04.001

Mystkowski, J. L., Mineka, S., Vernon, L. L., & Zinbarg, R. E. (2003). Changes in caffeine states enhance return of fear in spider phobia. *Journal of Consulting and Clinical Psychology*, *71*(2), 243–250. https://doi.org/10.1037/0022–006X.71.2.243

Nacasch, N., Foa, E. B., Huppert, J. D., Tzur, D., Fostick, L., Dinstein, Y., Polliack, M., & Zohar, J. (2011). Prolonged exposure therapy for combat- and terror-related posttraumatic stress disorder: A randomized control comparison with treatment as usual. *Journal of Clinical Psychiatry*, *72*(9), 1174-1180. https://doi.org/10.4088/ JCP.09m05682blu

Nacasch, N., Huppert, J. D., Su, Y. J., Kivity, Y., Dinshtein, Y., Yeh, R., & Foa, E. B. (2015). Are 60-minute prolonged exposure sessions with 20-minute imaginal exposure to traumatic memories sufficient to successfully treat PTSD? A randomized noninferiority clinical trial. *Behavior Therapy, 46*(3), 328–341. https://doi.org/10.1016/j.beth.2014.12.002

Nam, D. H., Pae, C. U., & Chae, J. H. (2013). Low-frequency, repetitive transcranial magnetic stimulation for the treatment of patients with posttraumatic stress disorder: A double-blind, sham-controlled study. *Clinical Psychopharmological and Neuroscience, 11*, 96–102. https://doi.org/10.9758/cpn.2013.11.2.96

National Institute for Health and Care Excellence (NICE). (2018). *Guideline for posttraumatic stress disorder*. National Institute for Health and Clinical Practice.

Negreira, A. M., & Abdallah, C. G. (2019). A review of fMRI affective processing paradigms used in the neurobiological study of posttraumatic stress disorder. *Chronic Stress, 3*. https://doi.org/10.1177/2470547019829035

Newson, J. J., & Thiagarajan, T. C. (2019). EEG frequency bands in psychiatric disorders: A review of resting state studies. *Frontiers in Human Neuroscience, 12*(521), 521. Advance online publication. https://doi.org/10.3389/fnhum.2018.00521

Neylan, T. C., Brunet, A., Pole, N., Best, S. R., Metzler, T. J., Yehuda, R., & Marmar, C. R. (2005). PTSD symptoms predict waking salivary cortisol levels in police officers. *Psychoneuroendocrinology, 30*(4), 373–381. https://doi.org/10.1016/j.psyneuen.2004.10.005

Norman, S. B., Trim, R., Haller, M., Davis, B. C., Myers, U. S., Colvonen, P. J., Blanes, E., Lyons, R., Siegel, E. Y., Angkaw, A. C., Norman, G. J., & Mayes, T. (2019). Efficacy of integrated exposure therapy vs integrated coping skills therapy for comorbid posttraumatic stress disorder and alcohol use disorder. *JAMA Psychiatry, 76*, 791.

Norrholm, S. D., Glover, E. M., Stevens, J. S., Fani, N., Galatzer-Levy, I. R., Bradley, B., Ressler, K. J., & Jovanovic, T. (2015). Fear load: The psychophysiological over-expression of fear as an intermediate phenotype associated with trauma reactions. *International Journal of Psychophysiology, 98*(2), 270–275. https://doi.org/10.1016/j.ijpsycho.2014.11.005

Norrholm, S. D., & Jovanovic, T. (2018). Fear processing, psychophysiology, and PTSD. *Harvard Review of Psychiatry, 26*(3), 129–141. https://doi.org/10.1097/HRP.0000000000000189

Norrholm, S. D., Jovanovic, T., Gerardi, M., Breazeale, K. G., Price, M., Davis, M., Duncan, E., Ressler, K. J., Bradley, B., Rizzo, A., Tuerk, P. W., & Rothbaum, B. O. (2016). Baseline psychophysiological and cortisol reactivity as a predictor of PTSD treatment outcome in virtual reality exposure therapy. *Behaviour Research and Therapy, 82*, 28–37. https://doi.org/10.1016/j.brat.2016.05.002

Norrholm, S. D., Jovanovic, T., Olin, I. W., Sands, L. A., Karapanou, I., Bradley, B., & Ressler, K. J. (2011). Fear extinction in traumatized civilians with posttraumatic stress disorder: Relation to symptom severity. *Biological Psychiatry, 69*(6), 556–563. https://doi.org/10.1016/j.biopsych.2010.09.013

Norton, P. J., Hayes-Skelton, S. A., & Klenck, S. C. (2011). What happens in session does not stay in session: Changes within exposures predict subsequent improvement and dropout. *Journal of Anxiety Disorders, 25*(5), 654–660. https://doi.org/10.1016/j.janxdis.2011.02.006

Oehen, P., Traber, R., Widmer, V., & Schnyder, U. (2013). A randomized, controlled pilot study of MDMA ($\pm$ 3,4-methylenedioxymethamphetamine)-assisted psychotherapy for treatment of resistant, chronic post-traumatic stress disorder (PTSD). *Journal of Psychopharmacology, 27*(1), 40–52. https://doi.org/10.1177/0269881112464827

O'Kearney, R., & Perrott, K. (2006). Trauma narratives in posttraumatic stress disorder: A review. *Journal of Traumatic Stress, 19*, 81–93. https://doi.org/10.1002/jts.20099

Øktedalen, T., Hoffart, A., & Langkaas, T. F. (2015). Trauma-related shame and guilt as time-varying predictors of posttraumatic stress disorder symptoms during imagery exposure and imagery rescripting—A randomized controlled trial. *Psychotherapy Research, 25*(5), 518–532. https://doi.org/10.1080/10503307.2014.917217

Olff, M., de Vries, G. J., Güzelcan, Y., Assies, J., & Gersons, B. P. (2007). Changes in cortisol and DHEA plasma levels after psychotherapy for PTSD. *Psychoneuroendocrinology, 32*, 619–626. https://doi.org/10.1016/j.psyneuen.2007.04.001

Olff, M., Langeland, W., Witteveen, A., & Denys, D. (2010). A psychobiological rationale for oxytocin in the treatment of posttraumatic stress disorder. *CNS Spectrums, 15*(8), 522–530. https://doi.org/10.1017/S109285290000047X

Olff, M., & van Zuiden, M. (2017). Neuroendocrine and neuroimmune markers in PTSD: Pre-, peri- and post-trauma glucocorticoid and inflammatory dysregulation. *Current Opinion in Psychology, 14*, 132–137. https://doi.org/10.1016/j.copsyc.2017.01.001

Orcutt, H. K., Hannan, S. M., Seligowski, A. V., Jovanovic, T., Norrholm, S. D., Ressler, K. J., & McCanne, T. (2017). Fear-potentiated startle and fear extinction in a sample of undergraduate women exposed to a campus mass shooting. *Frontiers in Psychology, 7*(2031), 2031. Advance online publication. https://doi.org/10.3389/fpsyg.2016.02031

Oliver, N. S., & Page, A. C. (2003). Fear reduction during in vivo exposure to blood-injection stimuli: Distraction vs. attentional focus. *British Journal of Clinical Psychology, 42*(1), 13–25. https://doi.org/10.1348/014466503762841986

Orr, S. P., Lasko, N. B., Macklin, M. L., Pineles, S. L., Chang, Y., & Pitman, R. K. (2012). Predicting post-trauma stress symptoms from pre-trauma psychophysiologic reactivity, personality traits and measure of psychopathology. *Biology of Mood and Anxiety, 2*(8), 1–12. https://doi.org/10.1186/2045-5380-2-8

Orr, S. P., Metzger, L. J., Lasko, N. B., Macklin, M. L., Peri, T., & Pitman, R. K. (2000). De novo conditioning in trauma-exposed individuals with and without posttraumatic stress disorder. *Journal of Abnormal Psychology, 109*(2), 290–298. https://doi.org/10.1037/0021-843X.109.2.290

Orr, S. P., Pitman, R. K., Lasko, N. B., & Herz, L. R. (1993). Psychophysiological assessment of posttraumatic stress disorder imagery in World War II and Korean combat veterans. *Journal of Abnormal Psychology, 102*(1), 152–159. https://doi.org/10.1037/0021-843X.102.1.152

Osuch, E. A., Benson, B. E., Luckenbaugh, D. A., Geraci, M., Post, R. M., & McCann, U. (2009). Repetitive TMS combined with exposure therapy for PTSD: A preliminary study. *Journal of Anxiety Disorders, 23*(1), 54–59. https://doi.org/10.1016/j.janxdis.2008.03.015

Ouyang, M., Young, M. B., Lestini, M. M., Schutsky, K., & Thomas, S. A. (2012). Redundant catecholamine signaling consolidates fear memory via phospholipase C. *Journal of Neuroscience, 32*(6), 1932–1941. https://doi.org/10.1523/JNEUROSCI.5231-11.2012

Pacella, M. L., Feeny, N., Zoellner, L., & Delahanty, D. L. (2014). The impact of PTSD treatment on the cortisol awakening response. *Depression and Anxiety, 31*(10), 862–869. https://doi.org/10.1002/da.22298

Pan, X., Kaminga, A. C., Wen, S. W., & Liu, A. (2018). Catecholamines in post-traumatic stress disorder: A systematic review and meta-analysis. *Frontiers in Molecular Neuroscience, 11*, 450. https://doi.org/10.3389/fnmol.2018.00450

Paredes, D., & Morilak, D. A. (2019). A rodent model of exposure therapy: The use of fear extinction as a therapeutic intervention for PTSD. *Frontiers in Behavioral Neuroscience, 13*(46), 46. Advance online publication. https://doi.org/10.3389/fnbeh.2019.00046

Patel, R., Spreng, R. N., Shin, L. M., & Girard, T. A. (2012). Neurocircuitry models of posttraumatic stress disorder and beyond: A meta-analysis of functional neuroimaging studies. *Neuroscience and Biobehavioral Reviews, 36*(9), 2130–2142. https://doi.org/10.1016/j.neubiorev.2012.06.003

Paunovic, N., & Öst, L. G. (2001). Cognitive-behavior therapy vs exposure therapy in the treatment of PTSD in refugees. *Behaviour Research and Therapy, 39*(10), 1183–1197. https://doi.org/10.1016/S0005-7967(00)00093-0

Phelps, E. A., Delgado, M. R., Nearing, K. I., & Ledoux, J. E. (2004). Extinction learning in humans: Role of the amygdala and vmPFC. *Neuron, 43*(6), 897–905. https://doi.org/10.1016/j.neuron.2004.08.042

Philip, N. S., Barredo, J., Aiken, E., Larson, V., Jones, R. N., Shea, M. T., Greenberg, B. D., & van 't Wout-Frank, M. (2019). Theta-burst transcranial magnetic stimulation for posttraumatic stress disorder. *American Journal of Psychiatry, 176*(11), 939–948. https://doi.org/10.1176/appi.ajp.2019.18101160

Piaget, J. (1962). The stages of the intellectual development of the child. *Bulletin of the Menninger Clinic, 26*(3), 120–128.

Pineles, S. L., Nillni, Y. I., Pinna, G., Irvine, J., Webb, A., Arditte Hall, K. A., Hauger, R., Miller, M. W., Resick, P. A., Orr, S. P., & Rasmusson, A. M. (2018). PTSD in women is associated with a block in conversion of progesterone to the GABAergic neurosteroids allopregnanolone and pregnanolone measured in plasma. *Psychoneuroendocrinology, 93*, 133–141. https://doi.org/10.1016/j.psyneuen.2018.04.024

Pineles, S. L., Suvak, M. K., Liverant, G. I., Gregor, K., Wisco, B. E., Pitman, R. K., & Orr, S. P. (2013). Psychophysiologic reactivity, subjective distress, and their associations with PTSD diagnosis. *Journal of Abnormal Psychology, 122*(3), 635–644. https://doi.org/10.1037/a0033942

Pitman, R. K., Gilbertson, M. W., Gurvits, T. V., May, F. S., Lasko, N. B., Metzger, L. J., Shenton, M. E., Yehuda, R., Orr, S. P., & the Harvard/VA PTSD Twin Study Investigators. (2006). Clarifying the origin of biological abnormalities in PTSD through the study of identical twins discordant for combat exposure. *Annals of the New York Academy of Sciences, 1071*, 242–254. https://doi.org/10.1196/annals.1364.019

Pitman, R. K., Orr, S. P., Altman, B., Longpre, R. E., Poiré, R. E., & Macklin, M. L. (1996). Emotional processing during eye movement desensitization and reprocessing therapy of Vietnam veterans with chronic posttraumatic stress disorder. *Comprehensive Psychiatry, 37*(6), 419–429. https://doi.org/10.1016/S0010-440X(96)90025-5

Pitman, R. K., Orr, S. P., & Lasko, N. B. (1993). Effects of intranasal vasopressin and oxytocin on physiologic responding during personal combat imagery in Vietnam veterans with posttraumatic stress disorder. *Psychiatry Research, 48*(2), 107–117. https://doi.org/10.1016/0165-1781(93)90035-F

Pole, N. (2007). The psychophysiology of posttraumatic stress disorder: A meta-analysis. *Psychological Bulletin, 133*(5), 725–746. https://doi.org/10.1037/0033-2909.133.5.725

Popiel, A., Zawadzki, B., Pragłowska, E., & Teichman, Y. (2015). Prolonged exposure, paroxetine and the combination in the treatment of PTSD following a motor vehicle accident. A randomized clinical trial: The "TRAKT" study. *Journal of Behavior Therapy and Experimental Psychiatry, 48*, 17–26. https://doi.org/10.1016/j.jbtep.2015.01.002

Possemato, K., Kuhn, E., Johnson, E., Hoffman, J. E., Owen, J. E., Kanuri, N., De Stefano, L., & Brooks, E. (2016). Using PTSD Coach in primary care with and without clinician support: A pilot randomized controlled trial. *General Hospital Psychiatry, 38*, 94–98. https://doi.org/10.1016/j.genhosppsych.2015.09.005

Possemato, K., Ouimette, P., Lantinga, L. J., Wade, M., Coolhart, D., Schohn, M., & Strutynski, K. (2011). Treatment of Department of Veterans Affairs primary care patients with posttraumatic stress disorder. *Psychological Services, 8*(2), 82–93. https://doi.org/10.1037/a0022704

Power, K., McGoldrick, T., Brown, K., Buchanan, R., Sharp, D., Swanson, V., & Karatzias, A. (2002). A controlled comparison of eye movement desensitization and reprocessing versus exposure plus cognitive restructuring versus waiting list in the treatment of post-traumatic stress disorder. *Clinical Psychology & Psychotherapy, 9*(5), 299–318.

Powers, M. B., Halpern, J. M., Ferenschak, M. P., Gillihan, S. J., & Foa, E. B. (2010). A meta-analytic review of prolonged exposure for posttraumatic stress disorder. *Clinical Psychology Review, 30*(6), 635–641. https://doi.org/10.1016/j.cpr.2010.04.007

Powers, M. B., Medina, J. L., Burns, S., Kauffman, B. Y., Monfils, M., Asmundson, G. J. G., Diamond, A., McIntyre, C., & Smits, J. A. (2015). Exercise augmentation of exposure therapy for PTSD: Rationale and pilot efficacy data. *Cognitive Behaviour Therapy, 44*(4), 314–327. https://doi.org/10.1080/16506073.2015.1012740

Prasad, A., Chaichi, A., Kelley, D. P., Francis, J., & Gartia, M. R. (2019). Current and future functional imaging techniques for post-traumatic stress disorder. *RSC Advances, 9*(42), 24568–24594. https://doi.org/10.1039/C9RA03562A

Price, M., Gros, D. F., Strachan, M., Ruggiero, K. J., & Acierno, R. (2013). The role of social support in exposure therapy for Operation Iraqi Freedom/Operation Enduring Freedom veterans: A preliminary investigation. *Psychological Trauma: Theory, Research, Practice, and Policy, 5*(1), 93–100. https://doi.org/10.1037/a0026244

Rabe, S., Zoellner, T., Beauducel, A., Maercker, A., & Karl, A. (2008). Changes in brain electrical activity after cognitive behavioral therapy for posttraumatic stress disorder in patients injured in motor vehicle accidents. *Psychosomatic Medicine, 70*(1), 13–19. https://doi.org/10.1097/PSY.0b013e31815aa325

Rabinak, C. A., Angstadt, M., Lyons, M., Mori, S., Milad, M. R., Liberzon, I., & Phan, K. L. (2014). Cannabinoid modulation of prefrontal-limbic activation during fear extinction learning and recall in humans. *Neurobiology of Learning and Memory, 113*, 125–134. https://doi.org/10.1016/j.nlm.2013.09.009

Rabinak, C. A., Angstadt, M., Sripada, C. S., Abelson, J. L., Liberzon, I., Milad, M. R., & Phan, K. L. (2013). Cannabinoid facilitation of fear extinction memory recall in humans. *Neuropharmacology, 64*, 396–402. https://doi.org/10.1016/j.neuropharm.2012.06.063

Rabinak, C. A., Peters, C., Elrahal, F., Milad, M., Rauch, S., Phan, L., & Greenwald, M. (2018). Cannabinoid facilitation of fear extinction in posttraumatic stress disorder. *Biological Psychiatry, 83*(9), S21. https://doi.org/10.1016/j.biopsych.2018.02.069

Ragsdale, K. A., & Voss Horrell, S. C. (2016). Effectiveness of prolonged exposure and cognitive processing therapy for US Veterans with a history of traumatic brain injury. *Journal of Traumatic Stress, 29*(5), 474–477.

Raskind, M. A., Peskind, E. R., Chow, B., Harris, C., Davis-Karim, A., Holmes, H. A., Hart, K. L., McFall, M., Mellman, T. A., Reist, C., Romesser, J., Rosenheck, R., Shih, M. C., Stein, M. B., Swift, R., Gleason, T., Lu, Y., & Huang, G. D. (2018). Trial of prazosin for post-traumatic stress disorder in military veterans. *New England Journal of Medicine, 378*(6), 507–517. https://doi.org/10.1056/NEJMoa1507598

Rasmussen, K. G. (2015). Ketamine for posttraumatic stress disorder. *JAMA Psychiatry, 72*(1), 94–95. https://doi.org/10.1001/jamapsychiatry.2014.1621

Rasmusson, A. M., King, M. W., Valovski, I., Gregor, K., Scioli-Salter, E., Pineles, S. L., Hamouda, M., Nillni, Y. I., Anderson, G. M., & Pinna, G. (2019). Relationships between cerebrospinal fluid GABAergic neurosteroid levels and symptom severity in men with PTSD. *Psychoneuroendocrinology, 102*, 95–104. https://doi.org/10.1016/j.psyneuen.2018.11.027

Rasmusson, A. M., & Pineles, S. L. (2018). Neurotransmitter, peptide, and steroid hormone abnormalities in PTSD: Biological endophenotypes relevant to treatment. *Current Psychiatry Reports, 20*, 52. https://doi.org/10.1007/s11920-018-0908-9

Rasmusson, A. M., Pinna, G., Paliwal, P., Weisman, D., Gottschalk, C., Charney, D., Krystal, J., & Guidotti, A. (2006). Decreased cerebrospinal fluid allopregnanolone levels in women with posttraumatic stress disorder. *Biological Psychiatry, 60*(7), 704–713. https://doi.org/10.1016/j.biopsych.2006.03.026

Rasmusson, A. M., Vasek, J., Lipschitz, D. S., Vojvoda, D., Mustone, M. E., Shi, Q., Gudmundsen, G., Morgan, C. A., Wolfe, J., & Charney, D. S. (2004). An increased capacity for adrenal DHEA release is associated with decreased avoidance and negative mood symptoms in women with PTSD. *Neuropsychopharmacology, 29*, 1546–1557. https://doi.org/10.1038/sj.npp.1300432

Rauch, S. A. M., Abelson, J. L., Javanbakht, A., & Liberzon, I. (2015). Neurobiology and translational approaches to posttraumatic stress disorder. In K. J. Ressler, D. J. Pine, & B. O. Rothbaum (Eds.), *Anxiety disorders: Translational perspectives on diagnosis and treatment* (pp. 121–134). Oxford University Press. https://doi.org/10.1093/med/9780199395125.003.0009

Rauch, S. A. M., Cigrang, J., Austern, D., Evans, A., & the STRONG STAR Consortium. (2017). Expanding the reach of effective PTSD treatment into primary care: Prolonged exposure for primary care. *Focus, 15*(4), 406–410. https://doi.org/10.1176/appi.focus.20170021

Rauch, S. A. M., & Foa, E. B. (2006). Emotional processing theory (EPT) and exposure therapy for PTSD. *Journal of Contemporary Psychotherapy, 36*(2), 61–65. https://doi.org/10.1007/s10879-006-9008-y

Rauch, S. A. M., Foa, E. B., Furr, J. M., & Filip, J. C. (2004). Imagery vividness and perceived anxious arousal in prolonged exposure treatment for PTSD. *Journal of Traumatic Stress, 17*(6), 461–465. https://doi.org/10.1007/s10960-004-5794-8

Rauch, S. A. M., Grunfeld, T. E., Yadin, E., Cahill, S. P., Hembree, E., & Foa, E. B. (2009). Changes in reported physical health symptoms and social function with prolonged exposure therapy for chronic posttraumatic stress disorder. *Depression and Anxiety, 26*(8), 732–738.

Rauch, S. A. M., Kim, H. M., Powell, C., Tuerk, P. W., Simon, N. M., Acierno, R., Allard, C. B., Norman, S. B., Venners, M. R., Rothbaum, B. O., Stein, M. B., Porter, K., Martis, B., King, A. P., Liberzon, I., Phan, K. L., & Hoge, C. W. (2019). Efficacy of prolonged exposure therapy, sertraline hydrochloride, and their combination among combat veterans with posttraumatic stress disorder: A randomized clinical trial. *JAMA Psychiatry, 76*(2), 117–126. https://doi.org/10.1001/jamapsychiatry.2018.3412

Rauch, S. A. M., King, A. P., Abelson, J., Tuerk, P. W., Smith, E., Rothbaum, B. O., Clifton, E., Defever, A., & Liberzon, I. (2015). Biological and symptom changes in posttraumatic stress disorder treatment: A randomized clinical trial. *Depression and Anxiety, 32*(3), 204–212. https://doi.org/10.1002/da.22331

Rauch, S. A. M., & Liberzon, I. (2016). Mechanisms of action in psychotherapy. In I. Liberzon & K. J. Ressler (Eds.) *Neurobiology of PTSD: From Brain to Mind*, (pp. 353–372). Oxford University Press.

Rauch, S. A. M., Simon, N. M., Kim, H. M., Acierno, R., King, A. P., Norman, S. B., Venners, M. R., Porter, K., Phan, K. L., Tuerk, P. W., Allard, C., Liberzon, I., Rothbaum, B. O., Martis, B., Stein, M. B., & Hoge, C. W. (2018). Integrating biological treatment mechanisms into randomized clinical trials: Design of PROGrESS (PROlonGed ExpoSure and Sertraline Trial). *Contemporary Clinical Trials, 64*, 128–138. https://doi.org/10.1016/j.cct.2017.10.013

Rauch, S. A. M., Sripada, R., Burton, M. B., Michopoulos, V., Kerley, K., Marx, C. E., Kilts, J. D., Naylor, J. C., Rothbaum, B. O., McLean, C. P, Smith, A., Norrholm, S. D., Jovanovic, T., Liberzon, I., Williamson, D., Yarvis, J. S., Dondanville, K. A., Young-McCaughan, S., Keane, T. M., Peterson, A. L., & the Consortium to Alleviate PTSD and the STRONG STAR Consortium. (2020a). Neuroendocrine biomarkers of prolonged exposure treatment response in military-related PTSD. *Psychoneuroendocrinology, 119*, Article 104749. https://doi.org/10.1016/j.psyneuen.2020.104749

Rauch, S. A. M., Sripada, R., Burton, M. B., Michopoulos, V., Kerley, K., Marx, C. E., Kilts, J. D., Naylor, J. C., Rothbaum, B. O., McLean, C. P, Smith, A., Norrholm, S. D., Jovanovic, T., Liberzon, I., Williamson, D., Yarvis, J. S., Dondanville, K. A., Young-McCaughan, S., Keane, T. M., Peterson, A. L., & the Consortium to Alleviate PTSD and the STRONG STAR Consortium. (2020b). Corrigendum to "Neuroendocrine biomarkers of prolonged exposure treatment response in military-related PTSD" [Psychoneuroendocrinology (2020a) Article 104749]. *Psychoneuroendocrinology, 120*, Article 104802. https://doi.org/10.1016/j.psyneuen.2020.104802

Rauch, S. A. M., Yasinski, C. W., Post, L. M., Jovanovic, T., Norrholm, S., Sherrill, A. M., Michopoulos, V., Maples-Keller, J. L., Black, K., Zwiebach, L., Dunlop, B. W., Loucks, L., Lannert, B., Stojek, M., Watkins, L., Burton, M., Sprang, K., McSweeney, L., Ragsdale, K., & Rothbaum, B. O. (2020). An intensive outpatient program with prolonged exposure for veterans with posttraumatic stress disorder: Retention, predictors, and patterns of change. *Psychological Services*. Advance online publication. https://doi.org/10.1037/ser0000422

Rauch, S. L., Shin, L. M., & Phelps, E. A. (2006). Neurocircuitry models of posttraumatic stress disorder and extinction: Human neuroimaging research—Past, present, and future. *Biological Psychiatry, 60*(4), 376–382. https://doi.org/10.1016/j.biopsych.2006.06.004

Rauch, S. L., Shin, L. M., Whalen, P. J., & Pitman, R. K. (1998). Neuroimaging and the neuroanatomy of posttraumatic stress disorder. *CNS Spectrums, 3*(S2), 30–41. https://doi.org/10.1017/S1092852900007306

Ready, D. J., Lamp, K., Rauch, S. A. M., Astin, M. C., & Norrholm, S. D. (2018). Extending prolonged exposure for veterans with posttraumatic stress disorder: When is enough really enough? *Psychological Services, 17*(2), 199–206. https://doi.org/10.1037/ser0000309

Reddy, D. S. (2010). Neurosteroids: Endogenous role in the human brain and therapeutic potentials. In I. Savic (Ed.), *Progress in brain research: Vol. 186. Sex differences in the human brain, their underpinnings and implications* (pp. 113–137). Elsevier Press.

Reger, G. M., Browne, K. C., Campellone, T. R., Simons, C., Kuhn, E., Fortney, J. C., & Reisinger, H. S. (2017). Barriers and facilitators to mobile application use during PTSD treatment: Clinician adoption of PE Coach. *Professional Psychology, Research and Practice, 48*(6), 510–517. https://doi.org/10.1037/pro0000153

Reger, G. M., Hoffman, J., Riggs, D., Rothbaum, B. O., Ruzek, J., Holloway, K. M., & Kuhn, E. (2013). The "PE coach" smartphone application: An innovative approach to improving implementation, fidelity, and homework adherence during prolonged exposure. *Psychological Services, 10*(3), 342–349. https://doi.org/10.1037/a0032774

Reger, G. M., Koenen-Woods, P., Zetocha, K., Smolenski, D. J., Holloway, K. M., Rothbaum, B. O., Difede, J., Rizzo, A. A., Edwards-Stewart, A., Skopp, N. A., Mishkind, M., Reger, M. A., & Gahm, G. A. (2016). Randomized controlled trial of prolonged exposure using imaginal exposure vs. virtual reality exposure in active duty soldiers with deployment-related posttraumatic stress disorder (PTSD). *Journal of Consulting and Clinical Psychology, 84*(11), 946–959. https://doi.org/10.1037/ccp0000134

Reger, G. M., Smolenski, D., Norr, A., Katz, A., Buck, B., & Rothbaum, B. O. (2019). Does virtual reality increase emotional engagement during exposure for PTSD? Subjective distress during prolonged and virtual reality exposure therapy. *Journal of Anxiety Disorders, 61*, 75–81. https://doi.org/10.1016/j.janxdis.2018.06.001

Rescorla, R. A., & Heth, C. D. (1975). Reinstatement of fear to an extinguished conditioned stimulus. *Journal of Experimental Psychology: Animal Behavior Processes, 1*(1), 88–96. https://doi.org/10.1037/0097-7403.1.1.88

Rescorla, R. A., & Wagner, A. R. (1972). *Classical conditioning: Current research and theory*. Appleton-Century-Crofts.

Resick, P. A., Galovski, T. E., Uhlmansiek, M. O. B., Scher, C. D., Clum, G. A., & Young-Xu, Y. (2008). A randomized clinical trial to dismantle components of cognitive processing therapy for posttraumatic stress disorder in female victims of interpersonal violence. *Journal of Consulting and Clinical Psychology, 76*(2), 243–258. https://doi.org/10.1037/0022-006X.76.2.243

Resick, P. A., Nishith, P., Weaver, T. L., Astin, M. C., & Feuer, C. A. (2002). A comparison of cognitive-processing therapy with prolonged exposure and a waiting condition for the treatment of chronic posttraumatic stress disorder in female rape victims. *Journal of Consulting and Clinical Psychology, 70*(4), 867–879. https://doi.org/10.1037/0022-006X.70.4.867

Resick, P. A., & Schnicke, M. K. (1993). *Cognitive processing therapy for rape victims: A treatment manual*. Newbury Park, CA: Sage.

Ressler, K. J., Mercer, K. B., Bradley, B., Jovanovic, T., Mahan, A., Kerley, K., Norrholm, S. D., Kilaru, V., Smith, A. K., Myers, A. J., Ramirez, M., Engel, A., Hammack, S. E.,

Toufexis, D., Braas, K. M., Binder, E. B., & May, V. (2011). Post-traumatic stress disorder is associated with PACAP and the PAC1 receptor. *Nature, 470*(7335), 492–497. https://doi.org/10.1038/nature09856

Ressler, K. J., Rothbaum, B. O., Tannenbaum, L., Anderson, P., Graap, K., Zimand, E., Hodges, L., & Davis, M. (2004). Cognitive enhancers as adjuncts to psychotherapy: Use of D-cycloserine in phobic individuals to facilitate extinction of fear. *Archives of General Psychiatry, 61*(11), 1136–1144. https://doi.org/10.1001/archpsyc.61.11.1136

Riha, P. D., Bruchey, A. K., Echevarria, D. J., & Gonzalez-Lima, F. (2005). Memory facilitation by methylene blue: Dose-dependent effect on behavior and brain oxygen consumption. *European Journal of Pharmacology, 511*(2–3), 151–158. https://doi.org/10.1016/j.ejphar.2005.02.001

Riley, W. T., McCormick, M. G. F., Simon, E. M., Stack, K., Pushkin, Y., Overstreet, M. M., Carmona, J. J., & Magakian, C. (1995). Effects of alprazolam dose on the induction and habituation processes during behavioral panic induction treatment. *Journal of Anxiety Disorders, 9*(3), 217–227. https://doi.org/10.1016/0887-6185(95)00003-7

Rizvi, S. L., Vogt, D. S., & Resick, P. A. (2009). Cognitive and affective predictors of treatment outcome in cognitive processing therapy and prolonged exposure for posttraumatic stress disorder. *Behaviour Research and Therapy, 47*(9), 737–743. https://doi.org/10.1016/j.brat.2009.06.003

Robison-Andrew, E. J., Duval, E. R., Nelson, C. B., Echiverri-Cohen, A., Giardino, N., Defever, A., Norrholm, S. D., Jovanovic, T., Rothbaum, B. O., Liberzon, I., & Rauch, S. A. (2014). Changes in trauma-potentiated startle with treatment of posttraumatic stress disorder in combat veterans. *Journal of Anxiety Disorders, 28*(4), 358–362. https://doi.org/10.1016/j.janxdis.2014.04.002

Rojas, J. C., Bruchey, A. K., & Gonzalez-Lima, F. (2012). Neurometabolic mechanisms for memory enhancement and neuroprotection of methylene blue. *Progress in Neurobiology, 96*(1), 32–45. https://doi.org/10.1016/j.pneurobio.2011.10.007

Rosenbaum, S., Sherrington, C., & Tiedemann, A. (2015). Exercise augmentation compared to usual care for post-traumatic stress disorder: A randomized controlled trial. *Acta Psychiatrica Scandinavica, 131*(5), 350–359.

Rosenfield, D., Smits, J. A. J., Hofmann, S. G., Mataix-Cols, D., de la Cruz, L. F., Andersson, E., Rück, C., Monzani, B., Pérez-Vigil, A., Frumento, P., Davis, M., de Kleine, R. A., Difede, J., Dunlop, B. W., Farrell, L. J., Geller, D., Gerardi, M., Guastella, A. J., Hendriks, G. J., . . . Otto, M. W. (2019). Changes in dosing and dose timing of D-cycloserine explain its apparent declining efficacy for augmenting exposure therapy for anxiety-related disorders: An individual participant-data meta-analysis. *Journal of Anxiety Disorders, 68*, 102149. https://doi.org/10.1016/j.janxdis.2019.102149

Rothbaum, B. O., Astin, M. C., & Marsteller, F. (2005). Prolonged exposure versus eye movement desensitization and reprocessing (EMDR) for PTSD rape victims. *Journal of Traumatic Stress, 18*(6), 607–616. https://doi.org/10.1002/jts.20069

Rothbaum, B. O., Cahill, S. P., Foa, E. B., Davidson, J. R., Compton, J., Connor, K. M., Astin, M. C., & Hahn, C. G. (2006). Augmentation of sertraline with prolonged exposure in the treatment of posttraumatic stress disorder. *Journal of Traumatic Stress, 19*(5), 625–638. https://doi.org/10.1002/jts.20170

Rothbaum, B. O., Price, M., Jovanovic, T., Norrholm, S. D., Gerardi, M., Dunlop, B., Davis, M., Bradley, B., Duncan, E. J., Rizzo, A., & Ressler, K. J. (2014). A randomized, double-blind evaluation of D-cycloserine or alprazolam combined with virtual reality exposure therapy for posttraumatic stress disorder in Iraq and Afghanistan War veterans. *American Journal of Psychiatry, 171*(6), 640–648. https://doi.org/10.1176/appi.ajp.2014.13121625

Rougemont-Bücking, A., Linnman, C., Zeffiro, T. A., Zeidan, M. A., Lebron-Milad, K., Rodriguez-Romaguera, J., Rauch, S. L., Pitman, R. K., & Milad, M. R. (2011). Altered processing of contextual information during fear extinction in PTSD: An fMRI study. *CNS Neuroscience & Therapeutics, 17*(4), 227–236. https://doi.org/10.1111/j.1755-5949.2010.00152.x

Rowe, M. K., & Craske, M. G. (1998). Effects of varied-stimulus exposure training on fear reduction and return of fear. *Behaviour Research and Therapy, 36*(7–8), 719–734. https://doi.org/10.1016/S0005-7967(97)10017-1

Ruglass, L. M., Shevorykin, A., Radoncic, V., Smith, K. M., Smith, P. H., Galatzer-Levy, I. R., Papini, S., & Hien, D. A. (2017). Impact of cannabis use on treatment outcomes among adults receiving cognitive-behavioral treatment for PTSD and substance use disorders. *Journal of Clinical Medicine, 6*(2), 14. https://doi.org/10.3390/jcm6020014

Ruwaard, J., Lange, A., Schrieken, B., & Emmelkamp, P. (2011). Efficacy and effectiveness of online cognitive behavioral treatment: A decade of interapy research. *Studies in Health Technology and Informatics, 167*, 9–14.

Sageman, S., & Brown, R. P. (2006). 3-acetyl-7-oxo-dehydroepiandrosterone for healing treatment-resistant posttraumatic stress disorder in women: 5 case reports. *Journal of Clinical Psychiatry, 67*, 493–496. https://doi.org/10.4088/JCP.v67n0323b

Salkovskis, P. M., Hackmann, A., Wells, A., Gelder, M. G., & Clark, D. M. (2007). Belief disconfirmation versus habituation approaches to situational exposure in panic disorder with agoraphobia: A pilot study. *Behaviour Research and Therapy, 45*, 877–885. https://doi.org/10.1016/j.brat.2006.02.008

Sander, L. B., Schorndanner, J., Terhorst, Y., Spanhel, K., Pryss, R., Baumeister, H., & Messner, E. M. (2020). "Help for trauma from the app stores?" A systematic review and standardised rating of apps for post-traumatic stress disorder (PTSD). *European Journal of Psychotraumatology, 11*(1), 1701–1788. https://doi.org/10.1080/20008198.2019.1701788

Sartory, G., Cwik, J., Knuppertz, H., Schürholt, B., Lebens, M., Seitz, R. J., & Schulze, R. (2013). In search of the trauma memory: A meta-analysis of functional neuroimaging studies of symptom provocation in posttraumatic stress disorder (PTSD). *PLOS ONE, 8*(3), e58150. https://doi.org/10.1371/journal.pone.0058150

Saunders, N., Downham, R., Turman, B., Kropotov, J., Clark, R., Yumash, R., & Szatmary, A. (2015). Working memory training with tDCS improves behavioral and neurophysiological symptoms in pilot group with post-traumatic stress disorder (PTSD) and with poor working memory. *Neurocase, 21*(3), 271–278. https://doi.org/10.1080/13554794.2014.890727

Scarpina, F., & Tagini, S. (2017). The Stroop color and word test. *Frontiers in Psychology, 8*(557), 557. Advance online publication. https://doi.org/10.3389/fpsyg.2017.00557

Schachter, S., & Singer, J. E. (1962). Cognitive, social, and physiological determinants of emotional state. *Psychological Review, 69*(5), 379–399. https://doi.org/10.1037/h0046234

Schmidt, U., & Vermetten, E. (2017). Integrating NIMH research domain criteria (RDoC) into PTSD research. *Current Topics in Behavioral Neurosciences, 38*, 69–91. https://doi.org/10.1007/7854_2017_1

Schneier, F. R., Neria, Y., Pavlicova, M., Hembree, E., Suh, E. J., Amsel, L., & Marshall, R. D. (2012). Combined prolonged exposure therapy and paroxetine for PTSD related to the World Trade Center attack: A randomized controlled trial. *American Journal of Psychiatry, 169*(1), 80–88. https://doi.org/10.1176/appi.ajp.2011.11020321

Schnurr, P. P., Friedman, M. J., Engel, C. C., Foa, E. B., Shea, M. T., Chow, B. K., Resick, P. A., Thurston, V., Orsillo, S. M., Haug, R., Turner, C., & Bernardy, N. (2007). Cognitive behavioral therapy for posttraumatic stress disorder in women: A randomized controlled trial. *Journal of the American Medical Association, 297*(8), 820–830. https://doi.org/10.1001/jama.297.8.820

Schür, R. R., Schijven, D., Boks, M. P., Rutten, B. P. F., Stein, M. B., Veldink, J. H., Joëls, M., Geuze, E., Vermetten, E., Luykx, J. J., & Vinkers, C. H. (2019). The effect of genetic vulnerability and military deployment on the development of posttraumatic stress disorder and depressive symptoms. *European Neuropsychopharmacology, 29*(3), 405–415. https://doi.org/10.1016/j.euroneuro.2018.12.009

Sharma, S., & Ressler, K. J. (2019). Genomic updates in understanding PTSD. *Progress in Neuro-Psychopharmacology & Biological Psychiatry, 90*, 197–203. https://doi.org/10.1016/j.pnpbp.2018.11.010

Shechner, T., Hong, M., Britton, J. C., Pine, D. S., & Fox, N. A. (2014). Fear conditioning and extinction across development: Evidence from human studies and animal models. *Biological Psychology, 100*, 1–12. https://doi.org/10.1016/j.biopsycho.2014.04.001

Sheerin, C. M., Lind, M. J., Bountress, K., Nugent, N. R., & Amstadter, A. B. (2017). The genetics and epigenetics of PTSD: Overview, recent advances, and future directions. *Current Opinion in Psychology, 14*, 5–11. https://doi.org/10.1016/j.copsyc.2016.09.003

Shemesh, E., Annunziato, R. A., Weatherley, B. D., Cotter, G., Feaganes, J. R., Santra, M., Yehuda, R., & Rubinstein, D. (2011). A randomized controlled trial of the safety and promise of cognitive–behavioral therapy using imaginal exposure in patients with posttraumatic stress disorder resulting from cardiovascular illness. *Journal of Clinical Psychiatry, 72*(2), 168–174. https://doi.org/10.4088/JCP.09m0511blu

Siette, J., Reichelt, A. C., & Westbrook, R. F. (2014). A bout of voluntary running enhances context conditioned fear, its extinction, and its reconsolidation. *Learning & Memory, 21*(2), 73–81. https://doi.org/10.1101/lm.032557.113

Simblett, S., Birch, J., Matcham, F., Yaguez, L., & Morris, R. (2017). A systematic review and meta-analysis of e-mental health interventions to treat symptoms of posttraumatic stress. *Journal of Medical Internet Research Mental Health, 4*(2), e14.

Simon, N. M., Connor, K. M., Lang, A. J., Rauch, S., Krulewicz, S., LeBeau, R. T., Davidson, J. R., Stein, M. B., Otto, M. W., Foa, E. B., & Pollack, M. H. (2008). Paroxetine CR augmentation for posttraumatic stress disorder refractory to prolonged exposure therapy. *Journal of Clinical Psychiatry, 69*, 400–405. https://doi.org/10.4088/JCP.v69n0309

Singewald, N., & Holmes, A. (2019). Rodent models of impaired fear extinction. *Psychopharmacology, 236*(1), 21–32. https://doi.org/10.1007/s00213-018-5054-x

Singewald, N., Schmuckermair, C., Whittle, N., Holmes, A., & Ressler, K. J. (2015). Pharmacology of cognitive enhancers for exposure-based therapy of fear, anxiety and trauma-related disorders. *Pharmacology & Therapeutics, 149*, 150–190. https://doi.org/10.1016/j.pharmthera.2014.12.004

Sloan, D. M., Lee, D. J., Litwack, S. D., Sawyer, A. T., & Marx, B. P. (2013). Written exposure therapy for veterans diagnosed with PTSD: A pilot study. *Journal of Traumatic Stress, 26*(6), 776–779. https://doi.org/10.1002/jts.21858

Sloan, D. M., Marx, B. P., Bovin, M. J., Feinstein, B. A., & Gallagher, M. W. (2012). Written exposure as an intervention for PTSD: A randomized clinical trial with motor vehicle accident survivors. *Behaviour Research and Therapy, 50*(10), 627–635. https://doi.org/10.1016/j.brat.2012.07.001

Sloan, D. M., Marx, B. P., Lee, D. J., & Resick, P. A. (2018). A brief exposure-based treatment vs cognitive processing therapy for posttraumatic stress disorder: A randomized noninferiority clinical trial. *JAMA Psychiatry, 75*(3), 233–239. https://doi.org/10.1001/jamapsychiatry.2017.4249

Sloan, T., & Telch, M. J. (2002). The effects of safety-seeking behavior and guided threat reappraisal on fear reduction during exposure: An experimental investigation. *Behaviour Research and Therapy, 40*(3), 235–251. https://doi.org/10.1016/S0005-7967(01)00007-9

Smith, E. R., Duax, J. M., & Rauch, S. A. M. (2013). Perceived perpetration during traumatic events: Clinical suggestions from experts in prolonged exposure therapy. *Cognitive and Behavioral Practice, 20*(4), 461–470.

Smoller, J. W. (2016). The genetics of stress-related disorders: PTSD, depression, and anxiety disorders. *Neuropsychopharmacology, 41*(1), 297–319. https://doi.org/10.1038/npp.2015.266

Smoller, J. W. (2019). Psychiatric genetics begins to find its footing. *American Journal of Psychiatry, 176*(8), 609–614. https://doi.org/10.1176/appi.ajp.2019.19060643

Soudry, Y., Lemogne, C., Malinvaud, D., Consoli, S. M., & Bonfils, P. (2011). Olfactory system and emotion: Common substrates. *European Annals of Otorhinolaryngology, Head and Neck Diseases, 128*(1), 18–23. https://doi.org/10.1016/j.anorl.2010.09.007

Spence, J., Titov, N., Solley, K., Dear, B. F., Johnston, L., Wootton, B., Kemp, A., Andrews, G., Zou, J., Lorian, C., & Choi, I. (2011). Characteristics and treatment preferences of people with symptoms of posttraumatic stress disorder: An internet survey. *PLOS ONE, 6*(7), e21864. https://doi.org/10.1371/journal.pone.0021864

Spoormaker, V. I., & Montgomery, P. (2008). Disturbed sleep in post-traumatic stress disorder: Secondary symptom or core feature? *Sleep Medicine Reviews, 12*(3), 169–184. https://doi.org/10.1016/j.smrv.2007.08.008

Sripada, R. K., Blow, F. C., Rauch, S. A. M., Ganoczy, D., Hoff, R., Harpaz-Rotem, I., & Bohnert, K. M. (2019). Examining the nonresponse phenomenon: Factors associated with treatment response in a national sample of veterans undergoing residential PTSD treatment. *Journal of Anxiety Disorders, 63*, 18–25. https://doi.org/10.1016/j.janxdis.2019.02.001

Sripada, R. K., King, A. P., Garfinkel, S. N., Wang, X., Sripada, C. S., Welsh, R. C., & Liberzon, I. (2012). Altered resting-state amygdala functional connectivity in men with posttraumatic stress disorder. *Journal of Psychiatry & Neuroscience, 37*(4), 241–249. https://doi.org/10.1503/jpn.110069

Sripada, R. K., & Rauch, S. A. (2015). Between-session and within-session habituation in prolonged exposure therapy for posttraumatic stress disorder: A hierarchical linear modeling approach. *Journal of Anxiety Disorders, 30*, 81–87. https://doi.org/10.1016/j.janxdis.2015.01.002

Sripada, R. K., Rauch, S. A. M., Tuerk, P. W., Smith, E., Defever, A. M., Mayer, R. A., Messina, M., & Venners, M. (2013). Mild traumatic brain injury and treatment response in prolonged exposure for PTSD. *Journal of Traumatic Stress, 26*(3), 369–375.

Sripada, R. K., Ready, D. J., Ganoczy, D., Astin, M. C., & Rauch, S. A. M. (2020). When to change the treatment plan: An analysis of diminishing returns in VA patients undergoing prolonged exposure and cognitive processing therapy. *Behavior Therapy, 51*, 85–98.

Stalder, T., Kirschbaum, C., Kudielka, B. M., Adam, E. K., Pruessner, J. C., Wüst, S., Dockray, S., Smyth, N., Evans, P., Hellhammer, D. H., Miller, R., Wetherell, M. A., Lupien, S. J., & Clow, A. (2016). Assessment of the cortisol awakening response: Expert consensus guidelines. *Psychoneuroendocrinology, 63*, 414–432. https://doi.org/10.1016/j.psyneuen.2015.10.010

Steenkamp, M. M., Litz, B. T., Hoge, C. W., & Marmar, C. R. (2015). Psychotherapy for military-related PTSD: A review of randomized clinical trials. *Journal of the American Medical Association, 314*(5), 489–500. https://doi.org/10.1001/jama.2015.8370

Stojek, M. M., McSweeney, L. B., & Rauch, S. A. M. (2018). Neuroscience informed prolonged exposure practice: Increasing efficiency and efficacy through mechanisms. *Frontiers in Behavioral Neuroscience, 12*, 281–281. https://doi.org/10.3389/fnbeh.2018.00281

Strawn, J. R., & Geracioti, T. D., Jr. (2008). Noradrenergic dysfunction and the psychopharmacology of posttraumatic stress disorder. *Depression and Anxiety, 25*(3), 260–271. https://doi.org/10.1002/da.20292

Stroud, L. R., Salovey, P., & Epel, E. S. (2002). Sex differences in stress responses: Social rejection versus achievement stress. *Biological Psychiatry, 52*(4), 318–327. https://doi.org/10.1016/S0006-3223(02)01333-1

Sun, L., Peräkylä, J., & Hartikainen, K. M. (2017). Frontal alpha asymmetry, a potential biomarker for the effect of neuromodulation on brain's affective circuitry-preliminary evidence from a deep brain stimulation study. *Frontiers in Human Neuroscience, 11*, 584–584. https://doi.org/10.3389/fnhum.2017.00584

Surís, A., North, C., Adinoff, B., Powell, C. M., & Greene, R. (2010). Effects of exogenous glucocorticoid on combat-related PTSD symptoms. *Annals of Clinical Psychiatry, 22*(4), 274–279. https://pubmed.ncbi.nlm.nih.gov/21180658

Szafranski, D. D., Smith, B. N., Gros, D. F., & Resick, P. A. (2017). High rates of PTSD treatment dropout: A possible red herring? *Journal of Anxiety Disorders, 47*, 91–98.

Tate, D. F., Shenton, M. E., & Bigler, E. D. (2012). Introduction to the brain imaging and behavior special issue on neuroimaging findings in mild traumatic brain injury. *Brain Imaging and Behavior, 6*(2), 103–107. https://doi.org/10.1007/s11682-012-9185-0

Taylor, S., Thordarson, D. S., Maxfield, L., Fedoroff, I. C., Lovell, K., & Ogrodniczuk, J. (2003). Comparative efficacy, speed, and adverse effects of three PTSD treatments: Exposure therapy, EMDR, and relaxation training. *Journal of Consulting and Clinical Psychology, 71*(2), 330–338. https://doi.org/10.1037/0022-006x.71.2.330

Telch, M. J., Bruchey, A. K., Rosenfield, D., Cobb, A. R., Smits, J., Pahl, S., & Gonzalez-Lima, F. (2014). Effects of post-session administration of methylene blue on fear extinction and contextual memory in adults with claustrophobia. *American Journal of Psychiatry, 171*(10), 1091–1098. https://doi.org/10.1176/appi.ajp.2014.13101407

Telch, M. J., Valentiner, D. P., Ilai, D., Young, P. R., Powers, M. B., & Smits, J. A. J. (2004). Fear activation and distraction during the emotional processing of claustrophobic fear. *Journal of Behavior Therapy and Experimental Psychiatry, 35*(3), 219–232. https://doi.org/10.1016/j.jbtep.2004.03.004

Thomaes, K., Dorrepaal, E., Draijer, N., Jansma, E. P., Veltman, D. J., & van Balkom, A. J. (2014). Can pharmacological and psychological treatment change brain structure and function in PTSD? A systematic review. *Journal of Psychiatric Research, 50,* 1–15. https://doi.org/10.1016/j.jpsychires.2013.11.002

Thorp, S. R., Glassman, L. H., Wells, S. Y., Walter, K. H., Gebhardt, H., Twamley, E., Golshan, S., Pittman, J., Penski, K., Allard, C., Morland, L. A., & Wetherell, J. (2019). A randomized controlled trial of prolonged exposure therapy versus relaxation training for older veterans with military-related PTSD. *Journal of Anxiety Disorders, 64,* 45–54. https://doi.org/10.1016/j.janxdis.2019.02.003

Tiet, Q. Q., Duong, H., Davis, L., French, R., Smith, C. L., Leyva, Y. E., & Rosen, C. (2019). PTSD coach mobile application with brief telephone support: A pilot study. *Psychological Services, 16*(2), 227–232. https://doi.org/10.1037/ser0000245

True, W. R., Rice, J., Eisen, S. A., Heath, A. C., Goldberg, J., Lyons, M. J., & Nowak, J. (1993). A twin study of genetic and environmental contributions to liability for posttraumatic stress symptoms. *Archives of General Psychiatry, 50*(4), 257–264. https://doi.org/10.1001/archpsyc.1993.01820160019002

Tsao, J. C. I., & Craske, M. G. (2000). Timing of treatment and return of fear: Effects of massed, uniform-, and expanding-spaced exposure schedules. *Behavior Therapy, 31*(3), 479–497. https://doi.org/10.1016/S0005-7894(00)80026-X

Tuerk, P. W., Wangelin, B. C., Powers, M. B., Smits, J. A. J., Acierno, R., Myers, U. S., Orr, S. P., Foa, E. B., & Hamner, M. B. (2018). Augmenting treatment efficiency in exposure therapy for PTSD: A randomized double-blind placebo-controlled trial of yohimbine HCl. *Cognitive Behaviour Therapy, 47*(5), 351–371. https://doi.org/10.1080/16506073.2018.1432679

Tuerk, P. W., Yoder, M., Ruggiero, K. J., Gros, D. F., & Acierno, R. (2010). A pilot study of prolonged exposure therapy for posttraumatic stress disorder delivered via telehealth technology. *Journal of Traumatic Stress, 23*(1), 116–123. https://doi.org/10.1002/jts.20494

Uddin, M., Chang, S.-C., Zhang, C., Ressler, K., Mercer, K. B., Galea, S., Keyes, K. M., McLaughlin, K. A., Wildman, D. E., Aiello, A. E., & Koenen, K. C. (2013). Adcyap1r1 genotype, posttraumatic stress disorder, and depression among women exposed to childhood maltreatment. *Depression and Anxiety, 30*(3), 251–258. https://doi.org/10.1002/da.22037

VA/DoD. (2017). *VA/DoD clinical practice guideline for the management of posttraumatic stress disorder and acute stress disorder.* U.S. Department of Veterans Affairs. https://www.healthquality.va.gov/guidelines/MH/ptsd/

Van Damme, S., Crombez, G., Hermans, D., Koster, E. H. F., & Eccleston, C. (2006). The role of extinction and reinstatement in attentional bias to threat: A conditioning approach. *Behaviour Research and Therapy, 44*(11), 1555–1563. https://doi.org/10.1016/j.brat.2005.11.008

van den Berg, D. P., de Bont, P. A., van der Vleugel, B. M., de Roos, C., de Jongh, A., Van Minnen, A., & van der Gaag, M. (2015). Prolonged exposure vs eye movement desensitization and reprocessing vs waiting list for posttraumatic stress disorder in patients with a psychotic disorder: A randomized clinical trial. *JAMA Psychiatry, 72*(3), 259–267.

van Minnen, A., Arntz, A., & Keijsers, G. P. J. (2002). Prolonged exposure in patients with chronic PTSD: Predictors of treatment outcome and dropout. *Behaviour Research and Therapy, 40*(4), 439–457. https://doi.org/10.1016/S0005-7967(01)00024-9

van Minnen, A., & Foa, E. B. (2006). The effect of imaginal exposure length on outcome of treatment for PTSD. *Journal of Traumatic Stress, 19*(4), 427–438. https://doi.org/10.1002/jts.20146

van Minnen, A., & Hagenaars, M. (2002). Fear activation and habituation patterns as early process predictors of response to prolonged exposure treatment in PTSD. *Journal of Traumatic Stress, 15*(5), 359–367. https://doi.org/10.1023/A:1020177023209

Van Voorhees, E. E., Dennis, M. F., Calhoun, P. S., & Beckham, J. C. (2014). Association of DHEA, DHEAS, and cortisol with childhood trauma exposure and post-traumatic stress disorder. *International Clinical Psychopharmacology, 29*(1), 56–62. https://doi.org/10.1097/YIC.0b013e328364ecd1

van Zuiden, M., Frijling, J. L., Nawijn, L., Koch, S. B. J., Goslings, J. C., Luitse, J. S., Biesheuvel, T. H., Honig, A., Veltman, D. J., & Olff, M. (2017). Intranasal oxytocin to prevent posttraumatic stress disorder symptoms: A randomized controlled trial in emergency department patients. *Biological Psychiatry, 81*(12), 1030–1040. https://doi.org/10.1016/j.biopsych.2016.11.012

Vogel, S., & Schwabe, L. (2016). Learning and memory under stress: Implications for the classroom. *NPJ: Science of Learning, 1*(1), 16011. https://doi.org/10.1038/npjscilearn.2016.11

Wachtel, S. R., ElSohly, M. A., Ross, S. A., Ambre, J., & de Wit, H. (2002). Comparison of the subjective effects of Delta(9)-tetrahydrocannabinol and marijuana in humans. *Psychopharmacology, 161*, 331–339. https://doi.org/10.1007/s00213-002-1033-2

Wahbeh, H., & Oken, B. S. (2013). Peak high-frequency HRV and peak alpha frequency higher in PTSD. *Applied Psychophysiology and Biofeedback, 38*(1), 57–69. https://doi.org/10.1007/s10484-012-9208-z

Wallace, A. E., Weeks, W. B., Wang, S., Lee, A. F., & Kazis, L. E. (2006). Rural and urban disparities in health-related quality of life among veterans with psychiatric disorders. *Psychiatric Services, 57*(6), 851–856. https://doi.org/10.1176/ps.2006.57.6.851

Walsh, K., Nugent, N. R., Kotte, A., Amstadter, A. B., Wang, S., Guille, C., Acierno, R., Kilpatrick, D. G., & Resnick, H. S. (2013). Cortisol at the emergency room rape visit as a predictor of PTSD and depression symptoms over time. *Psychoneuroendocrinology, 38*(11), 2520–2528. https://doi.org/10.1016/j.psyneuen.2013.05.017

Wang, T., Liu, J., Zhang, J., Zhan, W., Li, L., Wu, M., Huang, H., Zhu, H., Kemp, G. J., & Gong, Q. (2016). Altered resting-state functional activity in posttraumatic stress disorder: A quantitative meta-analysis. *Scientific Reports, 6*(1), 27131. https://doi.org/10.1038/srep27131

Wang, Y., Karstoft, K.-I., Nievergelt, C. M., Maihofer, A. X., Stein, M. B., Ursano, R. J., Bybjerg-Grauholm, J., Bækvad-Hansen, M., Hougaard, D. M., Andreassen, O. A., Werge, T., Thompson, W. K., & Andersen, S. B. (2019). Post-traumatic stress following military deployment: Genetic associations and cross-disorder genetic correlations. *Journal of Affective Disorders, 252*, 350–357. https://doi.org/10.1016/j.jad.2019.04.070

Wangelin, B. C., & Tuerk, P. W. (2015). Taking the pulse of prolonged exposure therapy: Physiological reactivity to trauma imagery as an objective measure of treatment response. *Depression and Anxiety, 32*(12), 927–934. https://doi.org/10.1002/da.22449

Watson, J. P., & Marks, I. M. (1971). Relevant and irrelevant fear in flooding: A crossover study of phobic patients. *Behavior Therapy, 2*(3), 275–293. https://doi.org/10.1016/S0005-7894(71)80062-X

Watts, B. V., Landon, B., Groft, A., & Young-Xu, Y. (2012). A sham controlled study of repetitive transcranial magnetic stimulation for posttraumatic stress disorder. *Brain Stimulation, 5*(1), 38–43. https://doi.org/10.1016/j.brs.2011.02.002

Weisman, J. S., & Rodebaugh, T. L. (2018). Exposure therapy augmentation: A review and extension of techniques informed by an inhibitory learning approach. *Clinical Psychology Review, 59*, 41–51. https://doi.org/10.1016/j.cpr.2017.10.010

Wessel, J. R. (2012). Error awareness and the error-related negativity: Evaluating the first decade of evidence. *Frontiers in Human Neuroscience, 6*, 88. https://doi.org/10.3389/fnhum.2012.00088

Wilk, J. E., West, J. C., Duffy, F. F., Herrell, R. K., Rae, D. S., & Hoge, C. W. (2013). Use of evidence-based treatment for posttraumatic stress disorder in Army behavioral healthcare. *Psychiatry, 76*(4), 336–348. https://doi.org/10.1521/psyc.2013.76.4.336

Williams, M. T., Malcoun, E., Sawyer, B. A., Davis, D. M., Bahojb Nouri, L., & Bruce, S. L. (2014). Cultural adaptations of prolonged exposure therapy for treatment and prevention of posttraumatic stress disorder in African Americans. *Behavioral Sciences (Basel, Switzerland), 4*(2), 102–124. https://doi.org/10.3390/bs4020102

Wisco, B. E., Baker, A. S., & Sloan, D. M. (2016). Mechanisms of change in written exposure treatment of posttraumatic stress disorder. *Behavior Therapy, 47*(1), 66–74. https://doi.org/10.1016/j.beth.2015.09.005

Wisco, B. E., Marx, B. P., Wolf, E. J., Miller, M. W., Southwick, S. M., & Pietrzak, R. H. (2014). Posttraumatic stress disorder in the US veteran population: Results from the National Health and Resilience in Veterans Study. *Journal of Clinical Psychiatry, 75*(12), 1338–1346. https://doi.org/10.4088/JCP.14m09328

Wolf, E. J., Miller, M. W., Sullivan, D. R., Amstadter, A. B., Mitchell, K. S., Goldberg, J., & Magruder, K. M. (2018). A classical twin study of PTSD symptoms and resilience: Evidence for a single spectrum of vulnerability to traumatic stress. *Depression and Anxiety, 35*(2), 132–139. https://doi.org/10.1002/da.22712

Wolf, E. J., Mitchell, K. S., Koenen, K. C., & Miller, M. W. (2014). Combat exposure severity as a moderator of genetic and environmental liability to post-traumatic stress disorder. *Psychological Medicine, 44*(7), 1499–1509. https://doi.org/10.1017/S0033291713002286

Wolf, G. K., Kretzmer, T., Crawford, E., Thors, C., Wagner, H. R., Strom, T. Q., Eftekhari, A., Klenk, M., Hayward, L., & Vanderploeg, R. D. (2015). Prolonged exposure therapy with veterans and active duty personnel diagnosed with PTSD and traumatic brain injury. *Journal of Traumatic Stress, 28*(4), 339–347.

Wolpe, J. (1954). Reciprocal inhibition as the main basis of psychotherapeutic effects. *A.M.A. Archives of Neurology and Psychiatry, 72*(2), 205–226. https://doi.org/10.1001/archneurpsyc.1954.02330020073007

Woon, F. L., & Hedges, D. W. (2009). Amygdala volume in adults with posttraumatic stress disorder: A meta-analysis. *Journal of Neuropsychiatry Clinical Neuroscience, 21*(1), 5–12. https://doi.org/10.1176/appi.neuropsych.21.1.5 10.1176/jnp.2009.21.1.5

Wright, K. D., Hickman, R., & Laudenslager, M. L. (2015). Hair cortisol analysis: A promising biomarker of HPA activation in older adults. *Gerontologist, 55*(Suppl. 1), S140–S145. https://doi.org/10.1093/geront/gnu174

Wrubel, K. M., Riha, P. D., Maldonado, M. A., McCollum, D., Gonzalez-Lima, F. (2007). The brain metabolic enhancer methylene blue improves discrimination learning in rats. *Pharmacology, Biochemistry and Behavior, 86*(4), 712–717.

Yasinski, C., Sherrill, A. M., Maples-Keller, J. L., Rauch, S. A. M., & Rothbaum, B. O. (2018). Intensive outpatient prolonged exposure for PTSD in post 9-11 veterans and service members: Program structure and preliminary outcomes of the Emory Healthcare Veterans Program. *Trauma Psychology News, 12*(3), 1–3.

Yehuda, R., Bierer, L. M., Pratchett, L. C., Lehrner, A., Koch, E. C., Van Manen, J. A., Flory, J. D., Makotkine, I., & Hildebrandt, T. (2015). Cortisol augmentation of a psychological treatment for warfighters with posttraumatic stress disorder: Randomized trial showing improved treatment retention and outcome. *Psychoneuroendocrinology, 51*, 589–597. https://doi.org/10.1016/j.psyneuen.2014.08.004

Yehuda, R., Bierer, L. M., Pratchett, L., & Malowney, M. (2010). Glucocorticoid augmentation of prolonged exposure therapy: Rationale and case report. *European Journal of Psychotraumatology, 1*, 5643. Advance online publication. https://doi.org/10.3402/ejpt.v1i0.5643

Yehuda, R., Halligan, S. L., Golier, J. A., Grossman, R., & Bierer, L. M. (2004). Effects of trauma exposure on the cortisol response to dexamethasone administration in PTSD and major depressive disorder. *Psychoneuroendocrinology, 29*(3), 389–404. https://doi.org/10.1016/S0306-4530(03)00052-0

Yehuda, R., Pratchett, L. C., Elmes, M. W., Lehrner, A., Daskalakis, N. P., Koch, E., Makotkine, I., Flory, J. D., & Bierer, L. M. (2014). Glucocorticoid-related predictors and correlates of post-traumatic stress disorder treatment response in combat veterans. *Interface Focus, 4*(5), 20140048-20140048. https://doi.org/10.1098/rsfs.2014.0048

Yuan, H., Phillips, R., Wong, C. K., Zotev, V., Misaki, M., Wurfel, B., Krueger, F., Feldner, M., & Bodurka, J. (2018). Tracking resting state connectivity dynamics in veterans with PTSD. *NeuroImage: Clinical, 19*, 260–270. https://doi.org/10.1016/j.nicl.2018.04.014

Yuen, E. K., Gros, D. F., Price, M., Zeigler, S., Tuerk, P. W., Foa, E. B., & Acierno, R. (2015). Randomized controlled trial of home-based telehealth versus in-person prolonged exposure for combat-related PTSD in veterans: Preliminary results. *Journal of Clinical Psychology, 71*(6), 500–512. https://doi.org/10.1002/jclp.22168

Zalta, A. K., Gillihan, S. J., Fisher, A. J., Mintz, J., McLean, C. P., Yehuda, R., & Foa, E. B. (2014). Change in negative cognitions associated with PTSD predicts symptom reduction in prolonged exposure. *Journal of Consulting and Clinical Psychology, 82*(1), 171–175. https://doi.org/10.1037/a0034735

Zammit, S., Lewis, C., Dawson, S., Colley, H., McCann, H., Piekarski, A., Rockliff, H., & Bisson, J. (2018). Undetected post-traumatic stress disorder in secondary-care mental health services: Systematic review. *British Journal of Psychiatry*, *212*(1), 11–18. https://doi.org/10.1192/bjp.2017.8

Zannas, A. S., & Binder, E. B. (2014). Gene-environment interactions at the FKBP5 locus: Sensitive periods, mechanisms and pleiotropism. *Genes, Brain, and Behavior*, *13*(1), 25–37. https://doi.org/10.1111/gbb.12104

Zhang, K., Qu, S., Chang, S., Li, G., Cao, C., Fang, K., Olff, M., Wang, L., & Wang, J. (2017). An overview of posttraumatic stress disorder genetic studies by analyzing and integrating genetic data into genetic database PTSDgene. *Neuroscience and Biobehavioral Reviews*, *83*, 647–656. https://doi.org/10.1016/j.neubiorev.2017.08.021

Zhang, Y., Feng, B., Xie, J. P., Xu, F. Z., & Chen, J. (2011). Clinical study on treatment of the earthquake-caused post-traumatic stress disorder by cognitive-behavior therapy and acupoint stimulation. *Journal of Traditional Chinese Medicine*, *31*(1), 60–63. https://doi.org/10.1016/S0254-6272(11)60014-9

Zhu, X., Suarez-Jimenez, B., Lazarov, A., Helpman, L., Papini, S., Lowell, A., Durosky, A., Lindquist, M. A., Markowitz, J. C., Schneier, F., Wager, T. D., & Neria, Y. (2018). Exposure-based therapy changes amygdala and hippocampus resting-state functional connectivity in patients with posttraumatic stress disorder. *Depression and Anxiety*, *35*(10), 974–984. https://doi.org/10.1002/da.22816

Zhutovsky, P., Thomas, R. M., Olff, M., van Rooij, S. J. H., Kennis, M., van Wingen, G. A., & Geuze, E. (2019). Individual prediction of psychotherapy outcome in posttraumatic stress disorder using neuroimaging data. *Translational Psychiatry*, *9*(1), 326. https://doi.org/10.1038/s41398-019-0663-7

Zoellner, L. A., Roy-Byrne, P. P., Mavissakalian, M., & Feeny, N. C. (2019). Doubly randomized preference trial of prolonged exposure versus sertraline for treatment of PTSD. *American Journal of Psychiatry*, *176*(4), 287–296. https://doi.org/10.1176/appi.ajp.2018.17090995

Zoellner, L. A., Telch, M., Foa, E. B., Farach, F. J., McLean, C. P., Gallop, R., Bluett, E. J., Cobb, A., & Gonzalez-Lima, F. (2017). Enhancing extinction learning in posttraumatic stress disorder with brief daily imaginal exposure and methylene blue: A randomized controlled trial. *Journal of Clinical Psychology*, *78*(7), e782–e789.

Zuj, D. V., Palmer, M. A., Hsu, C. M. K., Nicholson, E. L., Cushing, P. J., Gray, K. E., & Felmingham, K. L. (2016). Impaired fear extinction associated with PTSD increases with hours-since-waking. *Depression and Anxiety*, *33*(3), 203–210. https://doi.org/10.1002/da.22463

Zukowska-Grojec, Z. (1995). Neuropeptide Y: A novel sympathetic stress hormone and more. *Annals of the New York Academy of Sciences*, *771*, 219–233. https://doi.org/10.1111/j.1749-6632.1995.tb44683.x

Index

About the Authors

Sheila A. M. Rauch, PhD, is a professor in the Department of Psychiatry and Behavioral Sciences at the Emory University School of Medicine and serves as deputy director of the Emory Healthcare Veterans Program and director of mental health research and program evaluation at the VA Atlanta Healthcare System. She has developed programs, conducted research, and provided treatment for posttraumatic stress disorder (PTSD) and anxiety disorders for over 20 years. She has led several PTSD treatment outcome and mechanisms trials and has been training providers in PTSD treatment since 2000. She has published scholarly articles, chapters, and books on anxiety disorders and PTSD, focusing on neurobiology and factors involved in the development, maintenance, and treatment of anxiety disorders and PTSD, psychosocial factors in medical settings, and the relationship between physical health and anxiety. She is an author of the second edition of the *Prolonged Exposure* (PE) manual as well as the manual for an intensive outpatient version of PE.

Carmen P. McLean, PhD, is a clinical psychologist in the dissemination and training division of the National Center for PTSD at the Palo Alto VA Healthcare System and a clinical associate professor (affiliate) at Stanford University. She is a certified prolonged exposure provider and supervisor. Dr. McLean has published over 100 scholarly articles and chapters on topics related to PTSD and anxiety. Her research aims to increase the reach of exposure therapy for PTSD by examining implementation barriers and using technology and condensed delivery of exposure to address barriers to treatment access.